Color Atlas
of
Common Oral Diseases

Graduation

Passed

Color Atlas
of
Common Oral Diseases

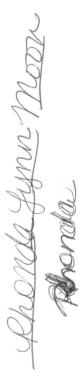

ROBERT P. LANGLAIS, DDS, MS

Professor, Department of Dental Diagnostic Science
University of Texas
Health Science Center
San Antonio, Texas

CRAIG S. MILLER, DMD, MS

Assistant Professor, Department of Oral Health Science
Oral Diagnosis Division
University of Kentucky
College of Dentistry
A.B. Chandler Medical Center
Lexington, Kentucky

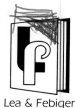

Lea & Febiger   Philadelphia/London

Williams & Wilkins
Rose Tree Corporate Center, Buildiing ll
1400 North Providence Road,Suite 5025
Media, PA 19063-2043 USA

Library of Congress Cataloging-in-Publication Data

Langlais, Robert P.
    Color atlas of common oral diseases/Robert P. Langlais, Craig S. Miller.
        p.   cm.
    The complete set of illustrations is also available for purchase as color slides.
    Includes index.
    ISBN 0-8121-1249-0
    1. Mouth–Diseases–Atlases.   2. Teeth–Diseases–Atlases.
I. Miller, Craig S.   II. Title
    [DNLM: 1. Mouth Diseases-pathology-atlases.   2. Tooth Diseases-pathology-atlases. WU
17 L282cl]
RC815.L36   1990
617.5′22′00222–dc20
DNLM/DLC
for Library of Congress   89-12561
                                                        CIP

Print number: 5

**To our wives,
Denyse and Sherry**

Foreword

Practicing oral medicine – that is, the diagnosis and treatment of oral manifestations of local or systemic diseases – is often a difficult challenge to the practitioner. This complexity stems from the many conditions that directly or indirectly affect the mouth and adjacent structures, and the entailing spectrum of signs and symptoms that often make a differential diagnosis quite difficult.

The organized approach that helps to simplify this aspect of oral health care delivery demands careful history taking, methodical oral examinations, recognition of normal structures and deviations from normal, and the capability of forming a differential diagnosis – a priority list of conditions or diseases that the findings suggest. The differential diagnosis forms the basis for performing tests that should lead to a definitive diagnosis and the appropriate treatment plan. These steps are important for standards of care, optimal patient health and function, protecting the clinician from censure, and to nurture meaningful referrals.

An important step of the diagnostic sequence, not to be overlooked, is the dental hygienist, who often sees the patient first. Since many signs and symptoms may represent malignancies, precancerous lesions, or infectious conditions, it is incumbent upon the dental hygienist to recognize deviations from normal, identify patients who may have these disorders, and inform the dentist of the clinical findings.

The Atlas by Drs Langlais and Miller greatly assists in the diagnostic process by providing an updated and organized approach to conditions that afflict the mouth. Chapters related to specific tissues, different sites, and clinical features of color and form are presented with a large number of high-quality color illustrations that have been carefully selected to represent features of conditions or diseases. The accompanying text is abbreviated to present concise overviews with emphasis on the clinical description of oral lesions, which allow a useful understanding of the entity in question. Available for use is a brief dictionary of useful terms that describes clinical findings, tables summarizing the characteristics of each group of disorders, and a separate listing of prescriptions useful in the management of these problems.

Since it is so difficult to master the complex variations of signs and symptoms associated with the multitude of oral manifestations of disease, a visual approach is one of the most helpful aids. Thus, this Atlas will be of significant help to clinicians at all levels of experience in creating a differential diagnosis, establishing a diagnosis, and forming a basis for a rational approach to managing and resolving patient problems.

SOL SILVERMAN, JR., M.A., D.D.S.

Preface

There are many excellent textbooks available of Oral Diagnosis, Oral Medicine, and Oral Pathology; however, after many years of our listening to requests by students for a high quality color atlas that is affordable, practical, and user-friendly, this publication has finally evolved. The goal of this color atlas is to provide both high-quality color illustrations and the salient clinical features of common oral diseases for those who are studying or attempting to identify oral disorders. The authors are fully aware that space has limited the scope of the written text, which is not intended to be all-inclusive, but rather to serve as a reference for the clinical diagnostic aspects of the more commonly encountered oral diseases. It is hoped that this text will be useful to students of dental assisting, dental hygiene, and dentistry by providing visual reinforcement of the written word. In addition, this book will be extremely useful to postgraduate dentists or hygienists whose goal is to become more knowledgeable about the clinical appearance of oral disease. This color atlas will also be of great value to practicing dentists, physicians, and specialists. Although many health-care providers may use this atlas as adjunctive material, the authors have made efforts to insure that the written material contained within is as current as possible. In this regard, the authors have extensively researched each disorder to insure that all statements are in concert with the current thinking of the majority of the profession.

The illustrations are arranged practically, according to clinical appearance, to facilitate the construction of a differential diagnosis. Each color plate consists of eight illustrations per page so that disorders closely related by appearance or etiology can be easily compared. For example, white lesions are grouped together, as are red lesions, ulcerative lesions, and so on. The illustrations selected for specific diseases have been chosen with the idea of showing each disorder in its most typical appearance and location. When several locations are possible, we have included several examples, often from the same patient. On the pages opposite the color plates, the written text discusses the nature of various disease processes, as well as other clinically relevant information such as location, sex, age, and race. The emphasis of the text is on the signs and symptoms of common oral diseases. Etiology and treatment methods are briefly discussed to provide additional valuable information. It is hoped that by arranging the material in this manner, the reader will be able to integrate concepts of oral diagnosis, oral medicine, oral pathology, and oral radiology.

Of some importance to all students of dentistry are a variety of helpful learning tips or methods. At the back of the text, the reader will find a glossary of terms, several tables of common oral conditions, prescriptions for the management of these disorders and a self-assessment test similar to those used in school examinations, state and national boards, and clinical sections of such speciality boards as Oral Medicine and Oral Pathology.

For those persons involved in education, the authors have the complete set of illustrations available for purchase as color slides. Details concerning the purchase of these slides are available by contacting:

Craig S. Miller, D.M.D., M.S.
MN 228, Division of Oral Diagnosis
University of Kentucky
College of Dentistry
Lexington, KY 40536-0084

San Antonio, Texas
Lexington, Kentucky

Robert P. Langlais
Craig S. Miller

Acknowledgments

We are extremely grateful to the many colleagues who have graciously provided material for publication in this atlas. Without their contributions, this fine quality text would not have been possible. We are also grateful to all practicing dentists and physicians who have referred patients throughout the years to the Department of Dental Diagnostic Science Referral Clinic.

To Professor Sol Silverman, who completely reviewed this text and wrote the foreword, we extend our thanks for his valuable comments and contributions. In addition, we are grateful for the many illustrations that Dr Silverman has provided, which can be seen throughout this text.

Dieter Karkut and Al Julian of the Photographic Services Section of Education Resources of The University of Texas Health Science Center receive a special thank you for their masterful job of cropping and recreating the proper color balance on our illustrations. We are especially grateful for the incredible efforts made by Dieter Karkut, who personally reviewed each color slide for possible color modifications and/or correction. We are also grateful to Albert Preciado and the entire Photography Unit, whose photography skills are evident throughout this work.

Finally, we would like to thank our wives, Denyse and Sherry, for their continuing support throughout this project. Authorship of a high quality text requires numerous off-duty hours; without the understanding and support of these two most important people in our lives, this work might never have been completed.

We also wish to express our appreciation to the following persons for contribution of their clinical photographs and radiographs used in this text.

Dr A. M. Abrams	Dr Marden Alder
Dr Tom Aufdemorte	Dr Bill Baker
Dr Douglas Barnett	Dr Pete Benson
Dr Howard Birkholz	Dr Steve Bricker
Dr Dale Buller	Dr Jerry Cioffi
Dr Laurie Cohen	Dr John Coke
Dr James Cottone	Dr Robert Craig, Jr
Dr S. Brent Dove	Dr David Freed
Dr Franklin Garcia-Godoy	Dr Birgit Glass
Dr Tom Glass	Dr Ed Heslop
Dr Micheal Huber	Dr Sheryl Hunter
Dr J. L. Jensen	Dr Ron Jorgenson
Dr Jerald Katz	Dr George Kaugers
Dr Olaf Langland	Dr Al Lugo
Dr Curt Lundeen	Dr Carson Mader
Dr Nancy Mantich	Dr Tom McDavid
Dr John McDowell	Dr Rick Myers
Dr Monique Michaud	Dr Dale Miles
Dr Charles Morris	Dr Chris Nortjé
Dr Linda Otis	Dr Roger Rao
Dr Tom Razmus	Dr Spencer Redding
Dr Michele Saunders	Dr Tom Schiff
Dr Jack Sherman	Dr Sol Silverman
Dr Larry Skoczylas	Dr D. B. Smith
Dr John Tall	Dr Geza Terezhalmy
Dr Martin Tyler	Dr Margot Van Dis
Dr Michael Vitt	Dr Elaine Winegard
Dr Donna Wood	

Contents

I

Diagnostic and Descriptive Terminology

DIAGNOSTIC AND DESCRIPTIVE TERMINOLOGY

Macule (Fig. 1-1) A macule is a circumscribed area of epidermis or mucosa distinguished by color from its surroundings. The macule may appear as a stain or spot that is blue, brown, or black in color. This lesion is neither elevated nor depressed and may be of any size. Most frequently the term "macule" is reserved for lesions 1 cm or smaller. The oral melanotic macule is an example of this condition.

Patch (Fig. 1-2) A patch is a circumscribed area that is larger than the macule and differentiated from the surrounding epidermis by color, or texture, or both. Like the macule, the patch is neither elevated nor depressed. Lichen planus, mucous patch of secondary syphilis, and snuff dipper's patch represent patch-like lesions that may be seen intraorally.

Erosion (Fig. 1-3) Erosion is a clinical term that describes a soft tissue lesion in which the epithelium above the basal cell layer is denuded. Erosions are moist, slightly depressed, and often result from a broken vesicle or trauma. Healing rarely results in scarring. Pemphigus is a disease that produces mucocutaneous erosions.

Ulcer (Fig. 1-4) An ulcer is an uncovered wound of cutaneous or mucosal tissue that exhibits gradual tissue disintegration and necrosis. Ulcers extend beyond the basal layer of the epithelium and into the dermis; thus scarring may follow healing. Ulcers may result from aphthous stomatitis, or infection by viruses such as herpes simplex, variola (smallpox), and varicella zoster (chickenpox and shingles). Ulcers are usually painful and often require topical drug therapy for effective management.

Wheal (Fig. 1-5) A wheal is an edematous papule or plaque that results from acute extravasation of serum into the upper dermis. Generally, wheals are pale red, pruritic, and of short duration; they often occur in allergic individuals. Wheals may be seen following insect bites, an allergic reaction to food, or mechanical irritation such as in patients who have dermatographia.

Scar (Fig. 1-6) A scar is a permanent mark or cicatrix remaining after a wound heals. These lesions are visible signs that indicate a disruption in the integrity of the epidermis and dermis. Scars are infrequently found in the oral cavity, but may be of any shape or size. The color of an intraoral scar is usually lighter than the adjacent mucosa. Periapical surgery or intraoral trauma may induce scar formation.

Fissure (Fig. 1-7) A fissure is a normal or abnormal linear cleft in the epidermis that typically affects the lips and perioral tissues. When pathogenic organisms infect a fissure pain, ulceration, and inflammation often result. Angular cheilitis and exfoliative cheilitis are examples of this condition.

Sinus (Fig. 1-8) A sinus is an abnormal tract or fistula that leads from a suppurative cavity, cyst, or abscess to the surface of the epidermis. An abscessed tooth often produces a sinus tract together with a clinically evident parulis, which is the terminal end of the sinus. Actinomycosis is a condition characterized by multiple sinus tracts that appear yellow in color.

DIAGNOSTIC AND DESCRIPTIVE TERMINOLOGY

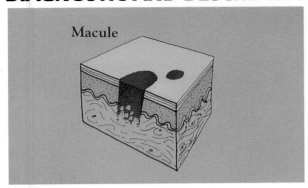

Fig. 1–1. Macule. A circumscribed area of epidermis altered in color from its surroundings.

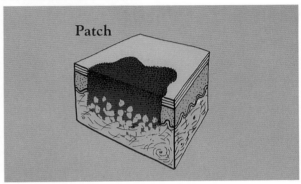

Fig. 1-2. Patch. A circumscribed pigmented or textured area larger than the macule.

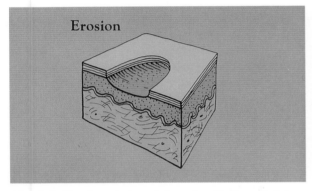

Fig. 1-3. Erosion. A denudation of epithelium above the basal cell layer.

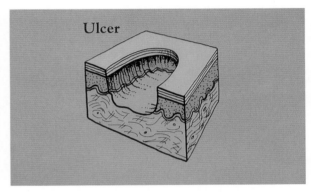

Fig. 1-4. Ulcer. A loss of epithelium that extends below the basal cell layer.

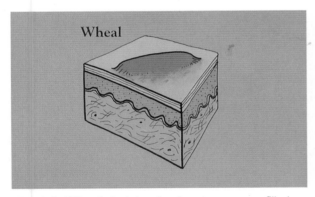

Fig. 1-5. Wheal. A pink-red, edematous, serum-filled papule or plaque.

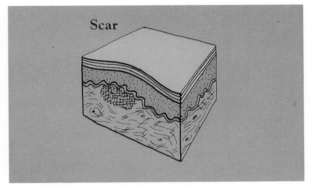

Fig. 1-6. Scar. A permanent mark indicative of previous wound healing.

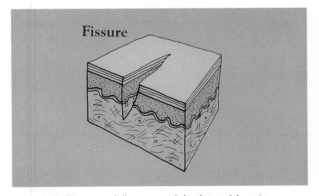

Fig. 1-7. Fissure. A linear crack in the epidermis.

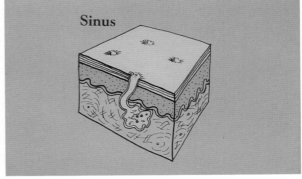

Fig. 1-8. Sinus. A tract leading from a suppurative cavity, cyst or abscess..

DIAGNOSTIC AND DESCRIPTIVE TERMINOLOGY

Papule (Fig. 2-1) A papule is a superficial, elevated, solid lesion that is smaller than 1 cm in diameter. Papules may be of any color and may be attached by a stalk or firm base. Examples of papules include the following conditions: condyloma acuminatum, parulis, and squamous papilloma.

Plaque (Fig. 2-2) A plaque is a flat, solid, raised area that is greater than 1 cm in diameter. Though essentially superficial, plaques may extend deeper into the dermis than papules. The edges may be sloped, and sometimes surface keratin proliferates, a condition known as lichenification. Lichen planus, leukoplakia or melanoma may initially appear as a plaque.

Nodule (Fig. 2-3) A nodule is a solid mass of tissue that has the dimension of depth. Like papules, these lesions are less than 1 cm in diameter, but nodules extend deeper into the dermis. Palpation provides detection of the nodule. The overlying epidermis is usually non-fixed and can be easily moved over the lesion. Benign mesenchymal tumors such as the fibroma, lipoma, lipofibroma, and neuroma often appear as oral nodules.

Tumor (Fig. 2-4) "Tumor" is a term used to represent a solid mass of tissue larger than 1 cm in diameter. The term is also used to represent a neoplasm – a new, independent growth of tissue with uncontrolled and progressive multiplication of cells that have no physiologic use. Tumors may be of any color and may be located in any intraoral soft tissue. Tumors often appear as raised rounded lesions that have the dimension of depth. Persistent tumors may be umbilicated or ulcerated in the center. The term tumor is often used to describe a benign tissue mass such as a neurofibroma, granular cell tumor, and pregnancy tumor.

Vesicle (Fig. 2-5) A vesicle is a circumscribed, fluid-filled elevation in the epidermis that is less than 1 cm in diameter. The fluid of a vesicle generally consists of lymph or serum, but may contain blood. The epithelial lining of a vesicle is thin and will eventually breakdown, thus giving rise to an ulcer and eschar. Vesicles are common in viral infections such as herpes simplex, herpes zoster, chickenpox, and smallpox.

Pustule (Fig. 2-6) A pustule is a circumscribed elevation filled with purulent exudate resulting from an infection. Pustules are less than 1 cm in diameter and may be preceded by a vesicle or papule. They appear creamy white or yellowish in color and are often associated with an epidermal pore. Intraorally the pustule is represented by a pointing abscess. Herpes zoster is another condition that produces pustules that eventually ulcerate and cause intense pain.

Bulla (Fig. 2-7) When a vesicle achieves a diameter greater than 1 cm, it is termed a bulla. This condition develops from the accumulation of fluid in the epidermal-dermis junction or a split in the epidermis. Bullae are commonly seen in pemphigus, pemphigoid, burns, and epidermolysis bullosa.

Cyst (Fig. 2-8) A cyst is an epithelially lined, often fluid-filled mass in the dermis or subcutaneous tissue. Cysts range in diameter from a few millimeters to several centimeters. Aspiration of a cyst may or may not yield luminal fluid, depending on the nature of the cyst. Cysts that contain clear fluid clinically appear pink to blue, whereas keratin-filled cysts often appear yellow or creamy white. There are many types of oral cysts. A small list includes the dermoid cyst, eruption cyst, implantation cyst, incisive canal cyst, lymphoepithelial cyst, mucous retention cyst, nasoalveolar cyst, and radicular cyst.

DIAGNOSTIC AND DESCRIPTIVE TERMINOLOGY

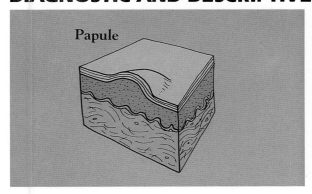

Fig. 2-1. Papule. An elevated, solid lesion less than 1 cm in diameter.

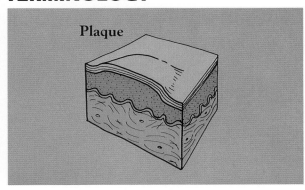

Fig. 2-2. Plaque. A flat, raised area greater than 1 cm in diameter.

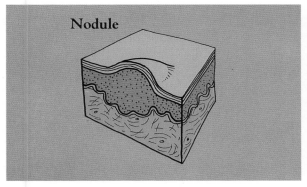

Fig. 2-3. Nodule. A raised, solid mass with the dimension of depth and is less than 1 cm in diameter.

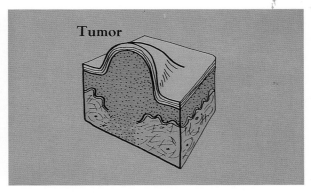

Fig. 2-4. Tumor. A solid, raised mass larger than 1 cm in diameter with the dimension of depth.

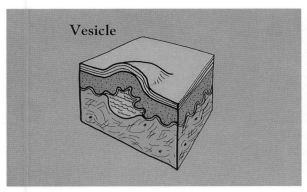

Fig. 2-5. Vesicle. A circumscribed, fluid-filled skin elevation less than 1 cm in diameter.

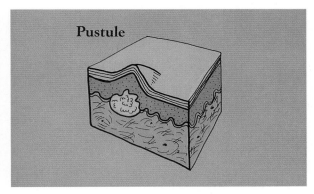

Fig. 2-6. Pustule. A vesicle filled with purulent exudate.

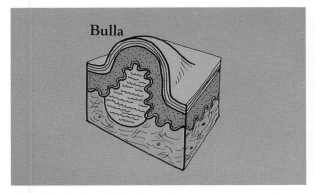

Fig. 2-7. Bulla. A fluid-filled skin elevation greater than 1 cm in diameter.

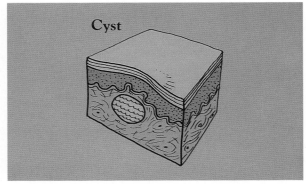

Fig. 2-8. Cyst. An epithelial lined, fluid-filled mass in the dermis or subcutaneous tissue.

Oral Conditions Affecting Infants and Children

ORAL CONDITIONS AFFECTING INFANTS AND CHILDREN

Congenital Epulis of the Newborn (Fig. 3-1)

The congenital epulis of the newborn is a soft tissue polypoid growth arising from the gingiva of the edentulous alveolar ridge of newborn infants. It usually occurs in the anterior maxilla, and is ten times more likely to occur in females than in males. The neoplasm is most likely of pericyte origin and histologically resembles a granular cell tumor. Clinically the lesion is pink, soft, and compressible. It usually attaches to the alveolar ridge by a pedunculated stalk and may reach several centimeters in diameter. Treatment is complete excision, and recurrence is unlikely.

Melanotic Neuroectodermal Tumor of Infancy (Fig. 3-2)

The melanotic neuroectodermal tumor of infancy is a benign, rapidly growing neuroblastic neoplasm commonly located in the anterior maxilla of infants less than 6 months old. The tumor shows no sexual predilection and begins as a small pink or red-purple nodule that resembles an eruption cyst. Localized and irregular destruction of underlying alveolar bone is the usual radiographic picture as well as a primary tooth bud floating in a soft tissue mass. Treatment is conservative excision. Histologic examination often reveals pigmentation. Recurrence and metastasis are rarely documented complications.

Dental Lamina Cysts (Fig. 3-3)

Remnants of the dental lamina that fail to develop into a tooth bud may degenerate to form dental lamina cysts. These cysts are classified, according to the clinical location in which they are found, as either Epstein's pearls or Bohn's nodules. Epstein's pearls are palatal keratin-filled cysts that develop from islands of epithelial cells that persist at the site of fusion of opposing embryonic palatal shelves. The pearls are usually small, firm, and whitish, and are found in groups of about three. They are usually located on the midline of the palate or at the junction of the hard and soft palates. Bohn's nodules, or gingival cysts, appear similar to Epstein's pearls, but are restricted to the alveolar ridge of infants. Dental lamina cysts vary in size from 1 mm to 1 cm, and both types are self-limiting. Resolution of Bohn's nodules occurs upon tooth eruption, whereas palatal cysts may be incised if they fail to resolve spontaneously.

Natal Teeth (Fig. 3-4)

Natal teeth are supernumerary odontogenic structures that appear occasionally in infants; most often as a familial trait. These predeciduous teeth are commonly located in the anterior mandible and frequently consist only of cornified and calcific material. Root formation is distinctly absent, and mobility is a common feature.

Natal teeth are believed to arise from an accessory tooth bud, and simple extraction is the recommended treatment. Natal teeth should be distinguished from a prematurely erupting deciduous tooth by taking the appropriate radiograph prior to dental treatment.

Gingival Eruption Cyst (Eruption Hematoma) (Fig. 3-5)

The eruption cyst is a soft tissue variant of the dentigerous cyst that forms around an erupting tooth crown. It is usually associated with primary teeth and manifests as a small, dome-shaped, bluish fluctuant swelling. The cyst is lined by odontogenic epithelium and filled with blood or serum. No treatment is usually necessary, as the erupting tooth will eventually break the cystic membrane. Symptomatic relief can be obtained by incising the lesion and allowing the fluid to drain.

Congenital Lymphangioma (Fig. 3-6)

The congenital lymphangioma is a benign neoplasm of dilated lymphatic channels that occasionally occurs within the mouth of infants. The tongue, labial mucosa, and alveolar ridge are common locations. No sexual predilection is evident. The lesion typically produces a swelling that is asymptomatic, compressible, and negative to diascopy. When superficial, the swelling is composed of single or multiple discrete papulonodules that may be pink to dark blue in color. Deep-seated tumors produce diffuse swellings with no alteration of the color of the overlying tissue. Large lymphangiomas of the neck are referred to as cystic hygromas. Surgical excision is the treatment of choice for intraoral lymphangiomas.

Thrush (Candidiasis, Moniliasis) (Fig. 3-7)

Thrush, or acute pseudomembranous candidiasis, is a fungal infection of mucosal membranes that is caused by *Candida albicans* and is primarily seen in infants. Thrush is a surface infection that produces milky-white curds on the oral mucosa. These curds are easily wiped off, leaving a red, raw, painful surface. The buccal mucosa, palate, and tongue are common locations of infection. Newborns often acquire the infection from the mother's birth canal during partuition and show clinical signs of disease within the first few weeks of life. Fever and gastrointestinal irritation may accompany the disorder. Treatment consists of antifungal agents applied topically.

Parulis (Gum Boil) (Fig. 3-8)

The parulis is an inflammatory response to a chronic bacterial infection of a non-vital tooth draining through a sinus tract. The condition is most common in children following the spread of pulpal infection to the furcal area of a posterior tooth. It clinically appears as a small, raised, fluctuant yellow-to-red boil that is located near the mucogingival junction adjacent to the affected tooth. Pressure to the area and the resulting discharge of pus is pathognomonic. Spontaneous pain is not a feature, although palpation of the lesion, tooth, or surrounding structures may elicit pain. Elimination of the odontogenic infection leads to resolution.

ORAL CONDITIONS AFFECTING INFANTS AND CHILDREN

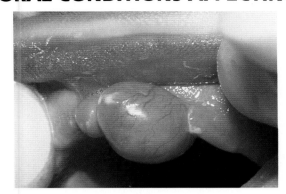

Fig. 3-1. Congenital epulis of the newborn. (Courtesy Dr Sheryl Hunter)

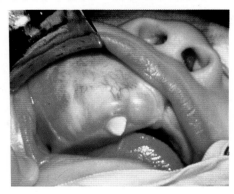

Fig. 3-2. Floating tooth in the **melanotic neuroectodermal tumor of infancy.** (Courtesy Dr Chris Nortjé)

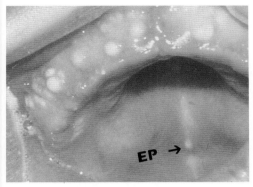

Fig. 3-3. Dental lamina cysts on the maxillary alveolar ridge and **epstein pearl** (EP) on median palatal raphe.

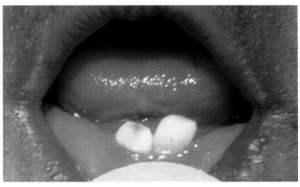

Fig. 3-4. Mandibular natal teeth. (Courtesy Dr Ron Jorgenson)

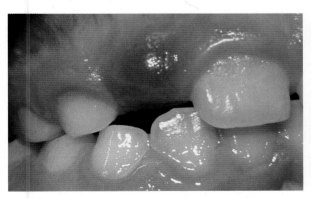

Fig. 3-5. Dome-shaped **gingival eruption cyst.** (Courtesy Dr F. Garcia-Godoy)

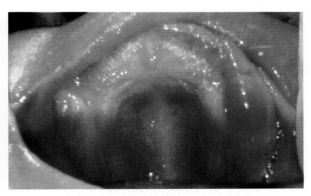

Fig. 3-6. Congenital alveolar lymphangioma. (Courtesy Dr Ron Jorgenson)

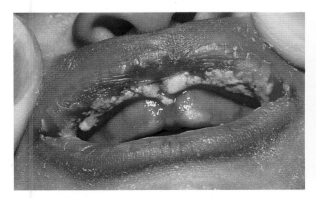

Fig. 3-7. Thrush caused by <u>Candida</u> <u>albicans</u>. (Courtesy Dr Ron Jorgenson)

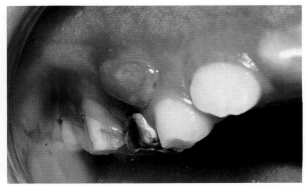

Fig. 3-8. Parulis; non-vital primary first molar. (Courtesy Dr Al Lugo)

Abnormalities by Anatomic Location

ALTERATIONS IN TOOTH MORPHOLOGY

Microdontia (Figs. 4-1 and 4-2) and Macrodontia
Microdontia refers to permanent teeth that are considerably smaller than normal. It usually occurs bilaterally and is often a familial trait. Microdontia may occur as an isolated finding, as a relative condition, or in a generalized pattern. The most common form occurs as an isolated finding involving a single permanent tooth, usually the maxillary lateral incisor. The term "peg lateral" is often used to describe this variant, because the tooth is cone- or peg-shaped. Third molars are the second-most frequently affected teeth.

When microdontia occurs in a generalized pattern it may be relative to the size of the jaws. True generalized microdontia is rare and occurs when the size of the jaws is normal and the actual tooth size is small. Generalized microdontia has been associated with pituitary dwarfism and cancer therapy during the formative stage of tooth development. True microdonts should be distinguished from small overretained primary teeth and examined for the presence of a frequently coexisting anomaly, the dens in dente (see Fig. 4-7).

Macrodontia is the opposite of microdontia and refers to an abnormal increase in tooth size. This condition may affect one, several or infrequently all teeth. It is usually a relative phenomenon. Macrodontia is often seen in incisors, in mandibular third molars, and in a developmental condition known as hemihypertrophy, in which the affected side is larger than the unaffected side. A single macrodont should be distinguished from fusion or gemination, a common finding of incisors and cuspids. True generalized macrodontia is rare and may be a result of pituitary gigantism.

Fusion (Figs. 4-3 and 4-4) and Gemination (Figs. 4-5 and 4-6) Fusion and gemination are opposite conditions that involve alterations in tooth morphology resulting from a developmental disturbance during tooth formation. In fusion the union of two tooth buds at the level of the dentin forms a single tooth. This condition is often hereditary, and it affects the primary teeth more commonly than the permanent teeth. Incisor teeth are the most frequently involved. Clinically one sees an enlarged crown, often with an extra cusp, a notch at the incisal edge, and a vertical groove of variable length in the enamel. Radiographically a single large root or two roots with separate pulp canals may be observed. In rare instances, a normal tooth bud fuses with a developing supernumerary tooth, thus greatly resembling gemination.

Gemination is the condition in which one tooth attempts to split in two. It appears as an incompletely divided or bifid tooth. The teeth most often affected are the primary mandibular incisors and permanent maxillary incisors. Heredity appears to be an important etiologic factor.

The two developmental anomalies, fusion and gemination, appear similar clinically and radiographically, and may be difficult to distinguish. Geminated teeth appear wide in the mesio-distal dimension, and more commonly lack the vertical groove that delineates the two crowns. To confirm the diagnosis the teeth should be counted. If a clinically large tooth is seen and there is no increase or decrease in tooth number, the condition is gemination. If an enlarged tooth is seen and a neighboring tooth is missing, fusion has occurred. Treatment is usually cosmetic, in which case the pulp chambers should be located radiographically prior to crown preparation or endodontic treatment.

Dens Invaginatus (Dens in Dente) (Fig. 4-7) and Dens Evaginatus (Leong's Tubercle) (Fig. 4-8) About 1% of the population has dens invaginatus, a developmental anomaly in which enamel and dentin of the crown invaginate in an apical direction into the pulp chamber along the palatal or lingual aspect of the tooth. There are various degrees of invagination and the term "dens in dente," which literally means a tooth within a tooth, should be reserved for only the most severe form of this disorder. Dens invaginatus is usually bilateral, and the cingulum of maxillary lateral incisors is the most frequent point of invagination, followed by the maxillary central incisors, mesiodens, cuspids, and mandibular lateral incisors. Clinically, the condition may appear as either a deep crevice or an accentuated lingual pit. Food can easily impact in the invagination, resulting in caries, which can rapidly lead to pulpal necrosis and periapical inflammation. Generally, prophylactic restorations are placed if the risk is high for carious involvement. Radiographically, one sees longitudinal and bulb-shaped layers of enamel, dentin, and pulp centrally located within the crown of the tooth. The disturbance may extend apically to involve the entire root.

Dens evaginatus is less common than dens invaginatus. It is represented by a small, dome-shaped accessory cusp emanating from either the central groove of the occlusal surface or the lingual incline of the buccal cusp of a permanent posterior tooth. This condition occurs almost exclusively in mandibular premolars, and as such has been termed Leong's tubercle. Persons of Mongolian descent exhibit Leong's tubercle more frequently than others. The tubercle consists of enamel, dentin, and a prominent pulp chamber. Care should be taken to prevent pulp injury during tooth preparation. Pathologic exposure of the pulp may occur with attrition.

ALTERATIONS IN TOOTH MORPHOLOGY

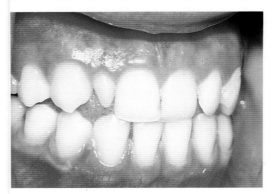

Fig. 4-1. **Microdontia;** peg-lateral incisor.

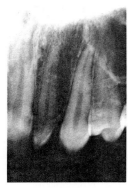

Fig. 4-2. Periapical radiograph of a **microdont** (peg lateral incisor).

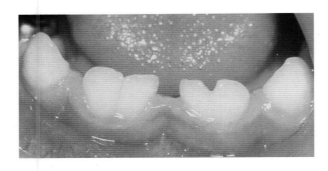

Fig. 4-3. Bilateral **fusion** of primary mandibular incisors. (Courtesy Dr Rick Myers)

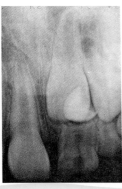

Fig. 4-4. Periapical radiograph of **fusion;** primary maxillary incisors.

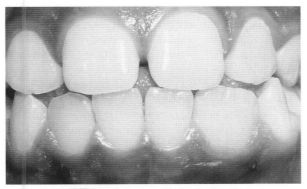

Fig. 4-5. **Gemination** of mandibular lateral incisor.

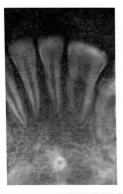

Fig. 4-6. Periapical radiograph of **gemination**.

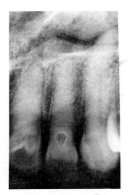

Fig. 4-7. Periapical radiograph of **dens invaginatus**.

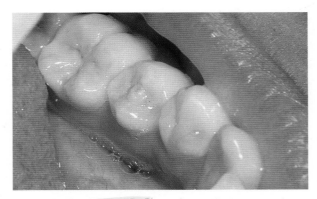

Fig. 4-8. **Dens evaginatus** of mandibular second premolar.

ALTERATIONS IN NUMBERS OF TEETH

Hypodontia (Figs. 5-1 and 5-2) Hypodontia is the congenital absence of one or a few teeth because of agenesis. Similar in meaning is the term oligodontia, which is used to refer to *numerous* congenitally missing teeth. The term anodontia is reserved for the rare condition involving the failure of all teeth to develop. When missing teeth are discovered, careful patient questioning is required to determine the reason for hypodontia. If teeth are missing for reasons such as prior removal or lack of eruption, the use of the term hypodontia is inappropriate.

Hypodontia may involve either sex, any race, and the primary or permanent teeth; however, it is most common in the permanent dentition. About 5% of the population is affected, and a familial tendency is quite common. The most frequent congenitally missing teeth are the third molars, followed by the mandibular second premolars, the maxillary second premolars, and the maxillary lateral incisors. Visible space or over-retained primary teeth are often the clinical signs of a missing tooth. Counting the teeth together with radiographs confirms the condition.

Many syndromes are associated with congenitally missing teeth. They include Böök's syndrome, chondroectodermal dysplasia, ectodermal dysplasia, incontinentia pigmenti, otodental dysplasia, and Rieger's syndrome. Both head and neck therapeutic radiation to infants or children and rubella (measles) during pregnancy have been implicated in the failure of tooth development.

Excess space is a sequela of missing teeth that may result in drifting, tipping, and supraeruption of adjacent or opposing teeth. Alterations in occlusion may require orthodontic and prosthodontic therapy to restore function and aesthetics.

Hyperdontia (Figs. 5-3 and 5-4) Hyperdontia is a term describing an extra or supernumerary deciduous or permanent tooth. It occurs approximately eight times more frequently in the maxilla than in the mandible, and most often in the permanent dentition. The most common supernumerary tooth is the mesiodens, which is located, either erupted or impacted, between the maxillary central incisors. It may be of normal size and shape, but is usually a small tooth with a conically shaped crown and short root.

The second most common supernumerary tooth is the maxillary fourth molar, which can be fully developed or microdontic in size. If the fourth molar is buccal or lingual to the erupted third molar, the term "paramolar" is used; if it is positioned behind the third molar, the term "distomolar" is used. Mandibular premolars are occasionally supernumerary.

Supernumerary teeth are usually afunctional and may cause inflammation, food impaction, interference with tooth eruption, as well as positional, aesthetic, and masticatory problems. In addition, impacted supernumerary teeth may give rise to dentigerous cysts. Because hyperdontia occurs in association with cleidocranial dysplasia and

Gardner's syndrome, investigations should be performed to rule out these disorders.

Cleidocranial Dysplasia (Figs. 5-5 and 5-6) Cleidocranial dysplasia is an autosomal dominant hereditary disturbance of unknown etiology. This syndrome affects women and men equally, and is usually discovered during childhood or early adolescence.

Cleidocranial dysplasia is a developmental disorder characterized by defective ossification of the clavicles and cranium together with oral and sometimes long bone disturbances. Prominent features include delayed closure of the frontal, parietal, and occipital fontanelles of the skull, short stature, broad shoulders, prominent frontal eminences with bossing, small paranasal sinuses, an underdeveloped maxilla with a high narrow palate, and relative prognathism of the mandible. The clavicles may be absent or underdeveloped, permitting hypermobility of the shoulders whereby patients can bring their shoulders together in front of the chest.

The oral changes are dramatic, particularly on the panoramic radiograph, which can lead to early diagnosis of the condition. There is prolonged retention of the primary dentition, numerous unerupted supernumerary teeth, especially in the premolar and molar areas, and delayed eruption of the permanent teeth. The permanent teeth are often short-rooted and lack cellular cementum, which may be the cause of the defective eruption pattern. Treatment is complex, requiring surgical and orthodontic considerations.

Gardner's Syndrome (Figs. 5-7 and 5-8) Gardner's syndrome is an autosomal dominant condition with prominent orofacial features characterized by hyperdontia, impacted supernumerary teeth, and jaw osteomas. In addition to these features, patients have multiple epidermal cysts, multiple dermoid tumors, and multiple intestinal polyps. The osteomas occur most frequently in the craniofacial skeleton, especially in the mandible and paranasal sinuses; however, osteomas of the long bones are possible. Maxillofacial radiographs often demonstrate numerous round osteomas and multiple diffuse enostoses that impart a cotton-wool appearance to the jaws. When superficial in the skin, these slow-growing tumors are clinically detectable as rock-hard nodules. The skin cysts (epidermoid, dermoid, or sebaceous) are smooth-surfaced lumps that are commonly located on the ventral and dorsal thorax. Lipomas, fibromas, leiomyomas, and/or desmoid tumors may accompany this disorder.

The most serious consideration of Gardner's syndrome are the multiple polyps that affect the colorectal mucosa. These intestinal polyps have an extremely high potential for malignant transformation, resulting in adenocarcinoma of the colon in nearly 100% of patients by the age of 40. Early recognition of the orofacial manifestations necessitates prompt referral to a gastroenterologist together with genetic counselling.

ALTERATIONS IN NUMBERS OF TEETH

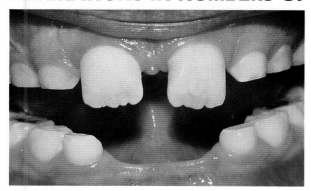

Fig. 5-1. Hypodontia; congenitally missing mandibular incisors.

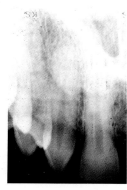

Fig. 5-2. Periapical radiograph revealing a congenitally missing maxillary lateral incisor; example of **hypodontia.**

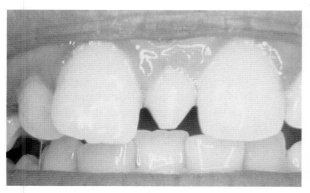

Fig. 5-3. Hyperdontia; fully erupted mesiodens.

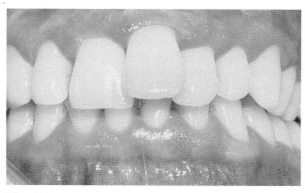

Fig. 5-4. Hyperdontia; extra maxillary lateral incisor.

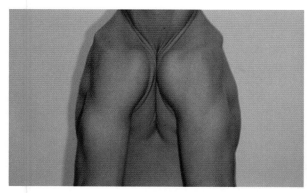

Fig. 5-5. Absent clavicles in a patient with **cleidocranial dysplasia.**

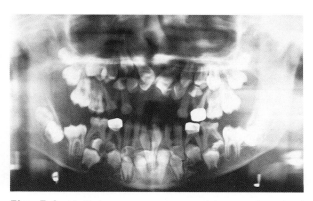

Fig. 5-6. Multiple supernumerary and impacted teeth of **cleidocranial dysplasia.**

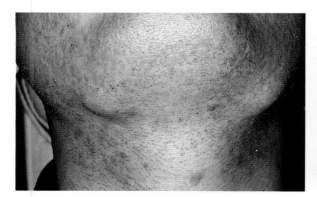

Fig. 5-7. Facial osteomas of **Gardner's syndrome.** (Courtesy Dr Geza Terezhalmy)

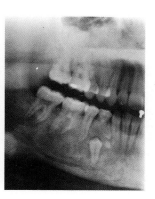
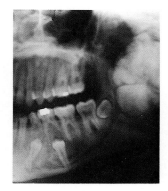

Fig. 5-8. Panoramic radiograph of a patient with **Gardner's syndrome.**

ALTERATIONS IN TOOTH STRUCTURE

Enamel Hypoplasia (Figs. 6-1 and 6-2) Enamel that is decreased in quantity is termed hypoplastic. This condition results from a disturbance in enamel deposition during amelogenesis. A variety of interfering influences, including genetic factors (amelogenesis imperfecta), local factors (trauma), or systemic factors (fluorosis, exanthematic microbial infections, and nutritional deficiencies), may be involved. Depending on the severity of hypoplasia enamel discolorations, surface pitting, or distinct horizontal grooves may appear. The pattern of enamel hypoplasia depends on the nature of the influencing factor, the phase of ameloblastic production at the time of the insult, and the duration of the insult. If the entire phase of amelogenesis is affected, the enamel of the entire dentition will be thin and may appear "snow-capped," yellowish-brown, rough, pitted, or mottled. If the influence is systemic and lasts only a short time, only enamel then being formed is affected, producing a linear band of hypocalcification on teeth developing during this period. If the injury is local, such as with trauma from an intruded primary tooth, damage to the labial enamel surface of the permanent successor is likely. Enamel hypoplasia of a single permanent tooth that results from periapical or perifurcal inflammation of a deciduous tooth is referred to as a "Turner's tooth."

Amelogenesis Imperfecta (Figs. 6-3 and 6-4) Amelogenesis imperfecta is a hereditary disorder that is characterized by a generalized defect in enamel formation of the primary and/or permanent dentition. The condition has been divided into four main types (hypoplastic, hypomature, hypocalcified, and hypomaturation-hypoplasia with taurodontism) and 11 subtypes according to clinical, histologic, radiographic, and genetic features.

The most common form, the hypoplastic type, is deficient in normal enamel, causing the crowns of the teeth to appear blanched, "snow-capped," yellow-brown, pitted, or grooved. Radiographically a full complement of teeth is usually seen; however, the crowns of the teeth demonstrate either very thin or absent enamel. The teeth resemble crown preparations with characteristic excessive interdental spacing.

The hypomature type has quantitatively normal amounts of enamel, but the enamel is soft and poorly mineralized; therefore a dental explorer under pressure will pit the enamel surface. In this type, the crowns contact interproximally but appear chalky, rough, grooved, and discolored. Fracturing of the enamel is common.

The hypocalcified type, like the hypomature type, has soft enamel but loses it at a much faster rate, resulting in exposed dentin soon after eruption. Patients with hypocalcified amelogenesis imperfecta usually have honey-colored teeth with roughened surface texture, multiple unerupted teeth, and an anterior open bite.

The hypomaturation-hypoplasia with taurodontism type exhibits yellowish teeth with opaque mottling, cervical pit-

ting, attrition, and taurodontism. Treatment for all forms of amelogenesis imperfecta is usually full veneer coverage for esthetic reasons.

Dentinogenesis Imperfecta (Figs. 6-5 and 6-6) Dentinogenesis imperfecta is a hereditary disorder that affects the development of dentin. Three types have been classified according to systemic involvement, clinical features, and histologic findings. They are Shields Type I, Shields Type II (hereditary opalescent dentin), and Shields Type III (Brandywine type).

Dentinogenesis imperfecta Shields Type I is a manifestation of osteogenesis imperfecta, a systemic condition involving bone fragility, blue sclerae, joint laxity, and hearing impairment. It is caused by a defect in collagen formation. Shields Type II demonstrates the same dentinal features as Type I, but no osteogenic component is present. Persons with Shields Type III have teeth that are opalescent in color like Types I and II, but the teeth have a shell-like appearance.

Dentinogenesis imperfecta affects the primary and permanent teeth, the latter less severely. Clinically, the teeth look normal when they first erupt, but shortly thereafter become discolored gray-brown or opalescent; the incisal and occlusal surfaces chip and flake away, resulting in fissuring and significant attrition. Radiographically one sees bulbous crowns, exaggerated cervical constrictions, short tapered roots, and progressive obliteration of the root canal. Affected teeth are more susceptible to root fractures.

Dentin Dysplasia (Figs. 6-7 and 6-8) Dentin dysplasia is a hereditary disorder of dentin characterized by alterations in pulp configuration – the presence of pulp stones, and idiopathic radiolucencies of the root apices. The term "rootless teeth" has been used to describe this condition. The abnormality has been classified into two types: Type I, radicular dentin dysplasia, and Type II, coronal dentin dysplasia. Both types are autosomal dominant and may affect the primary and permanent dentition.

The distinction between Types I and II is based on radiographic and histopathological findings. In Type I the primary and permanent teeth look clinically normal, but radiographs reveal defective root development with almost complete absence of root formation, as well as large pulp stones and complete pulpal obliteration of the primary teeth before tooth eruption. Loose teeth and multiple periapical radiolucencies of unknown etiology are characteristic.

In Type II the pulp canals of the primary teeth are often completely obliterated as they are with dentinogenesis imperfecta. The permanent teeth, in contrast, clinically appear normal except for narrower, thistle-shaped pulp canals that are frequently occupied by denticles. The roots may be short, blunted, and tapered, and may have horizontal radiolucent lines.

ALTERATIONS IN TOOTH STRUCTURE

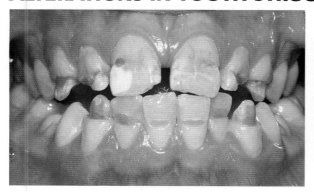

Fig. 6-1. Distinct grooves of **enamel hypoplasia.**

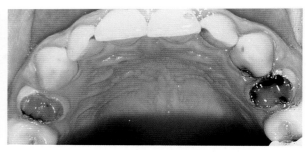

Fig. 6-2. Turner's teeth; maxillary first premolars.

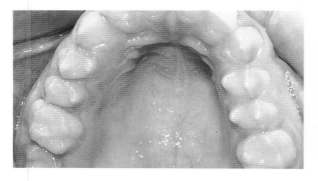

Fig. 6-3. Teeth of **amelogenesis imperfecta, hypoplastic type** that resembles crown preparations.

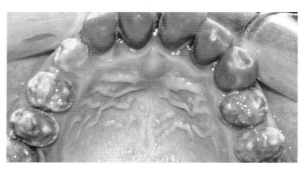

Fig. 6-4. Honey-colored teeth of **amelogenesis imperfecta, hypocalcified type.**

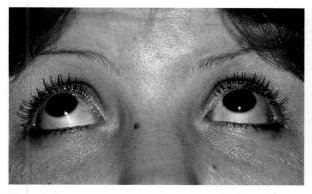

Fig. 6-5. Blue sclerae of **osteogenesis imperfecta Shields Type I.** (Courtesy Dr Jerald Katz)

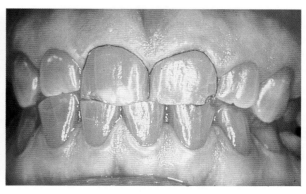

Fig. 6-6. Discolored teeth of **dentinogenesis imperfecta Shields Type I.** (Courtesy Dr Charles Morris)

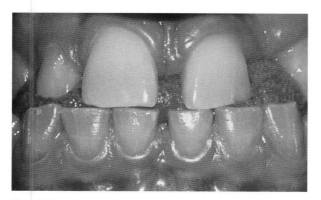

Fig. 6-7. Opalescent hue of teeth with **dentin dysplasia Type II.**

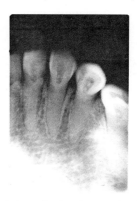

Fig. 6-8. Thistle-tube pulp chambers and pulp calcifications in the same patient with **dentin dysplasia** as in Fig. 6-7.

ACQUIRED DEFECTS OF TEETH

Caries *(Figs. 7-1 and 7-2)* Dental caries is one of the most common bacterial infections of man, characterized by demineralization and destruction of the organic matrix of teeth. Development of caries results from an interaction of bacterial plaque, diet components, altered host responses, and time. Electrochemical changes produced by acid generation and ion flow appear to be causative. The primary pathogen, *Streptococcus mutans*, together with *Actinomyces viscosus*, *Lactobacillus* species, and *Streptococcus sanguis* are closely involved in tooth adherence and the production of lactic acid necessary for the dissolution of enamel.

There are two types of caries, which are classified according to location: fissural and smooth surface. Fissural caries is the most common form. It occurs most often in deep fissures in the chewing surfaces of the posterior teeth. Smooth surface caries usually occurs at places that are protected from plaque removal such as just below the interproximal contact, at the gingival margin, and on the root surface.

Caries begins as an enamel decalcification that appears as a chalky white spot or fissure. A dental explorer tip is used to detect the soft lesion. Maturation of the lesion permits progression through the enamel, then laterally along the dentin-enamel junction, and eventually toward the pulp. Sensitivity to hot, cold, and sweets are usual symptoms; however, color changes, loss of hard tissue, or infection of the pulp may occur before the patient becomes aware of the disease. When caries occurs at an extremely rapid pace, as in some children and young adults, the term "rampant caries" is used. "Radiation, or amputation caries," is another form of caries that occurs in radiotherapy patients who lack the protective action of saliva. "Nursing bottle caries" is the result of prolonged contact of teeth with sugar-containing liquids in infants. "Root caries" are most frequently a result of xerostomia.

Pulp Polyp *(Fig. 7-3)* The pulp polyp is an inflammatory and hyperplastic response of a wide open pulp chamber to a chronic bacterial infection. Extensively carious deciduous molars and 6-year molars of young children are most frequently affected. Clinically the soft, red, nonpainful, pedunculated mass is seen projecting up from the pulp chamber beyond the broken-down occlusal surface of the tooth. Although the tooth is initially vital, the condition will eventually erode and result in nonvitality. Treatment is extraction or endodontic therapy.

Attrition *(Fig. 7-4)* Attrition, considered a physiologic process, is the loss of occlusal or incisal tooth structure due to chronic tooth-to-tooth frictional contact. Although the condition occurs most frequently in the elderly population, the primary teeth of young children may be affected. Attrition is usually a generalized condition accelerated by bruxism or abnormal use of selective teeth. Flattening of the interproximal region is a common sequela, whereas pulp exposure is a rare complication, since the deposition of secondary dentin and pulpal recession occur concurrently with the process. Close examination will reveal a smooth and highly polished tooth surface, the outline of the dentin-enamel junction, and the receded pulp chamber. Restoration of worn teeth may be challenging because of acquired changes in vertical dimension.

Abrasion *(Figs. 7-5 and 7-6)* Abrasion is the pathologic loss of tooth structure due to abnormal mechanical wear. A variety of agents can cause abrasion, but the most common form is "toothbrush abrasion," which produces a V-shaped notch in the cervical portion of the facial aspect of the tooth. The abraded area is usually shiny and yellow because of exposed dentin, and often the deepest portion of the groove is sensitive to the tine of the explorer. In addition to dentinal sensitivity, complications of abrasion are eventual pulp exposure or tooth fracture.

Abrasive notching of the teeth can be created by clasps of partial dentures, pins or nails habitually held with the teeth, or a pipe stem persistently clamped between the teeth. Abrasion of the incisal and occlusal surfaces often results from exposure to abrasive substances in the diet and occlusal wear from porcelain restorations placed in occlusion. The abrasive process is slow and chronic, requiring many years before giving rise to symptoms. Restoration of normal tooth contour may be unsuccessful if the patient is not made aware of the causative factors.

Erosion *(Figs. 7-7 and 7-8)* Erosion refers to the loss of tooth structure due to chemical action. Any chemical that is placed in prolonged contact with the tooth and produces a drop in pH can produce erosion. The labial and buccal surfaces of the teeth are most commonly affected.

The pattern of tooth erosion often indicates the causative agent or a particular habit. For example, lemon-sucking produces characteristic changes of the facial surfaces of the maxillary incisors. Horizontal ridges are initially apparent, followed by smooth, cupped-out, yellowish depressions. A similar erosive pattern may be seen in dedicated swimmers who chronically expose their anterior teeth to chlorinated swimming pools.

Erosion of the lingual surfaces of the maxillary teeth, together with amalgams that show generalized raised margins, may indicate chronic regurgitation due to bulimia, anorexia, pregnancy, or hiatal hernia. Sensitivity of the exposed area is an early symptom. Excessive consumption of sweetened carbohydrate beverages may accelerate the condition. Fluoride treatments for early erosions and restorations that cover exposed dentin for more extensive lesions are the treatment of choice. Habit elimination or behavior modification is required for success.

ACQUIRED DEFECTS OF TEETH

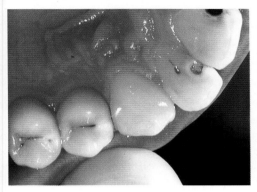

Fig. 7-1. Interproximal and occlusal **caries.**

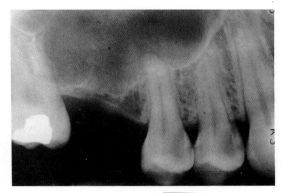

Fig. 7-2. Radiographic evidence of **caries** of same patient Fig. 7-1.

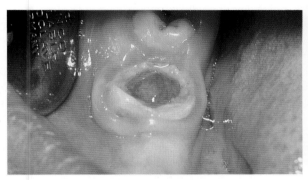

Fig. 7-3. Reddish, exuberant **pulp polyp** projecting up from the pulp chamber.

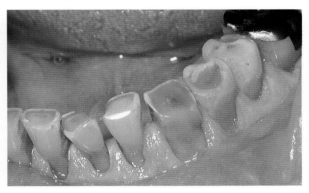

Fig. 7-4. Signs of **attrition**: smooth yellowish dentin exposed on masticatory surfaces.

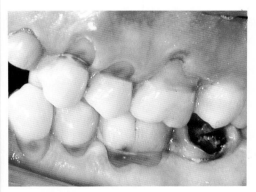

Fig. 7-5. Toothbrush abrasion along cervical margins of teeth.

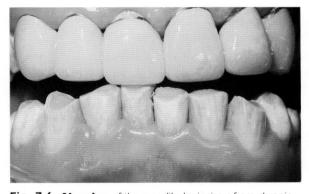

Fig. 7-6. Abrasion of the mandibular incisors from chronic friction against porcelain.

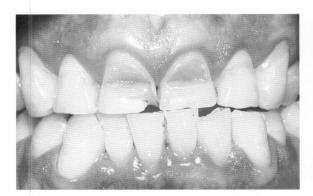

Fig. 7-7. Lemon-sucking erosion.

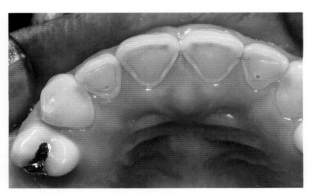

Fig. 7-8. Lingual **erosion of bulimia.**

LOCALIZED GINGIVAL LESIONS

Pyogenic Granuloma (Figs. 8-1 and 8-2) The term pyogenic granuloma is a misnomer, since it is neither pus-filled nor a granuloma; instead, it represents a form of inflammatory hyperplasia rich in neocapillaries and immature fibrous connective tissue. The exuberant growth is an exaggerated response to irritation and appears bright red, fleshy, and soft. The surface is glossy and the border is erythematous and ulcerated. The base may be polypoid or pedunculated. Although usually asymptomatic, minor manipulation will induce copious bleeding because of the thinned epithelium and highly vascular tissue. Maturation of the lesion results in increased fibrosis, decreased vascularity, and decreased intensity of color.

Pyogenic granulomas are prone to develop in patients who have poor oral hygiene or a chronic oral irritant such as overhanging restorations and calculus. Females are more susceptible to the condition because of hormonal influences. Pyogenic granulomas may correspond with hormonal imbalances that occur during puberty, pregnancy, or menopause, and in such cases are called "hormonal or pregnancy tumors." About 1% of pregnant women develop this lesion.

Pyogenic granulomas most frequently arise from the interdental papilla and enlarge from the labial and lingual aspects to several centimeters if left untreated. Other sites of development include the tongue, lips, buccal mucosa, and edentulous ridge. Treatment is surgical excision which, in the gravid female, should be delayed until after partuition. Recurrence is possible, especially if excision and local debridement are incomplete or if plaque control is inadequate.

Peripheral Giant Cell Granuloma (Figs. 8-3 and 8-4) The peripheral giant cell granuloma is a reactive epulis-like growth on the gingiva that is generally associated with a history of trauma or irritation. It is thought to originate from the mucoperiosteum or periodontal ligament; therefore, the peripheral giant cell granuloma demonstrates a restricted area of development – the dentulous or edentulous ridge. The mandibular gingiva anterior to the molars is particularly affected, especially in females between the ages of 10 and 40. Histologically multinucleated giant cells and fibroblasts are numerous throughout the specimen.

The peripheral giant cell granuloma is characterized by a well-defined, firm swelling that seldom ulcerates. The base is sessile, the surface is smooth or slightly granular, and the color is pink to dark red-purple. The nodule is usually a few millimeters to 1cm in diameter, although rapid enlargement may produce a large growth that encroaches on adjacent teeth. The lesion is generally asymptomatic, but because of its aggressive nature the underlying alveolar bone is often involved, producing a pathognomonic superficial "peripheral-cuff" radiolucency. Treatment is surgical excision including the base of the lesion and curettage of the underlying bone. Incomplete removal results in a marked tendency for recurrence. Histologically, this lesion cannot be distinguished from the central giant cell granuloma and the brown tumor of hyperparathyroidism.

Peripheral Fibroma with Calcification (Peripheral Cemento-Ossifying Fibroma) (Figs. 8-5 and 8-6) The etiology of the peripheral fibroma with calcification is uncertain, but inflammatory hyperplasia of superficial periodontal ligament origin has been suggested. It arises exclusively from the gingiva, usually the interdental papillae. When calcifications are present they may consist of bone, cementum, or dystrophic calcification, which are often difficult to distinguish microscopically.

The peripheral fibroma with calcification is a reactive growth that is especially prone to occur in the anterior region of the maxilla of young and middle-aged females. The salient clinical features of this solitary swelling are firmness, pink color, and sessile attachment. An important diagnostic clue is the condition's marked tendency to cause displacement of adjacent teeth. The chief complaint often involves an asymptomatic, slow-growing round or nodular swelling. Immature lesions are soft and bleed easily, whereas older lesions become firm and fibrotic. Radiographs may reveal central radiopaque foci and mild resorption of the crest of the ridge at its base. Treatment is excision. Care should be taken to avoid damage to the adjacent teeth. The recurrence rate is low.

Gingival Carcinoma (Figs. 8-7 and 8-8) The gingiva accounts for approximately 5 to 10% of all cases of squamous cell carcinoma within the mouth. Generally, at the time of diagnosis the disease is advanced because of its asymptomatic nature and posterior location, and because of delay of examination.

Gingival carcinoma has a varied appearance. It usually appears as a reddish mass with focal white areas proliferating from the gingiva, but may mimic benign inflammatory gingival conditions, erythroplakia, leukoplakia, or a simple ulceration. Carcinoma should be suspected when close examination reveals a pebbly surface, the presence of many small blood vessels in the overlying epithelium, and surface ulceration. Etiologic factors include tobacco use, alcoholism, and poor oral hygiene. Elderly males are especially susceptible, and the condition seems to have a slight predilection for the edentulous alveolar ridge of the posterior mandible. Completely dentulous persons rarely have this disease.

Gingival carcinoma may extend onto the floor of the mouth or mucobuccal fold, or it may invade the underlying bone. Radiographs may reveal a "cupping out" of the alveolar crest. Metastasis to regional lymph nodes occurs frequently. These nodes are firm, rubbery, matted, non-movable, and non-painful. Treatment consists of surgery and radiotherapy.

LOCALIZED GINGIVAL LESIONS

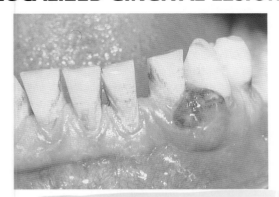

Fig. 8-1. **Pyogenic granuloma** arising from the interdental papilla.

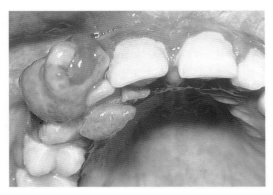

Fig. 8-2. **Pregnancy tumor;** three days post-partuition.

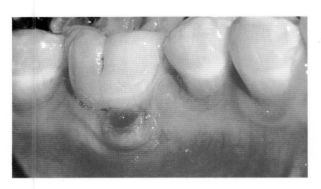

Fig. 8-3. Smooth-surfaced **peripheral giant-cell granuloma** arising from marginal gingiva. (Courtesy Dr Ed Heslop)

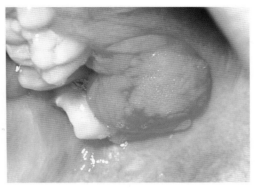

Fig. 8-4. A rapidly enlarging **peripheral giant-cell granuloma.** (Courtesy Drs James Cottone & Steve Bricker)

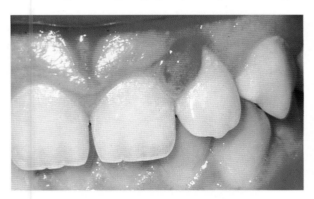

Fig. 8-5. **Peripheral fibroma with calcification** arising from the interdental papillae. (Courtesy Dr James Cottone)

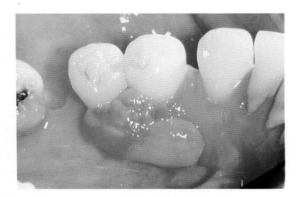

Fig. 8-6. Firm, pink **peripheral fibroma with calcification.** (Courtesy Dr Pete Benson)

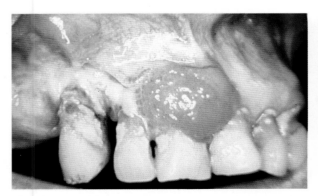

Fig. 8-7. **Gingival carcinoma** concurrent with poor oral hygiene and advanced age. (Courtesy Dr Jack Sherman)

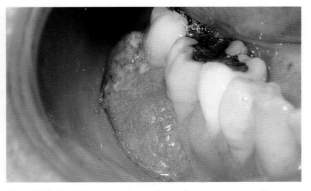

Fig. 8-8. Reddish, granular surface of **squamous cell carcinoma of the gingiva.** (Courtesy Dr Tom Aufdemorte)

LOCALIZED GINGIVAL LESIONS

Parulis (Gumboil) (Figs. 9-1 and 9-2) The parulis, or "gumboil" – a synonymous term reserved for children – is a localized area of inflammatory hyperplasia that occurs at the endpoint of a draining dental sinus tract. It appears as a soft, solitary reddish papule, located apical and facial to a chronically abscessed tooth, usually on or near the labial mucogingival junction. Occasionally the parulis is slightly yellow in the center and emits a purulent yellowish exudate upon palpation. Acute swelling and pain may accompany the condition if the sinus tract is obstructed.

To locate the non-vital tooth from which the parulis arises, a sterile gutta-percha point may be inserted into the fistula. Periapical radiographs are then taken to demonstrate the proximity of the gutta-percha point to the apex of the offending tooth. After diagnosing the non-vital tooth, the treatment of choice is root canal therapy. Regression of the parulis usually ensues shortly thereafter. If the problematic tooth is left untreated, the parulis may persist for years. A persistent lesion may mature into a pink-colored fibroma.

Pericoronitis (Operculitis) (Figs. 9-3 and 9-4) Pericoronitis is inflammation of the soft tissue surrounding the crown of a partially erupted or impacted tooth. Pericoronitis may develop at any age, but most frequently occurs in children and young adults whose teeth are erupting. Generally, it is associated with an erupting mandibular third molar that is in good alignment but is limited in its eruption by insufficient space. Radiographs of the region reveal a flame-shaped radiolucency surrounding the tooth, with the cortical outline on the distal aspect of the lucency either absent or distinctly thickened because of the deposition of reactive bone.

Pericoronitis develops from bacterial contamination beneath the operculum, resulting in gingival swelling, redness, and halitosis. The presence of pain is variable and may be extreme, but the discomfort usually resembles that of gingivitis, a periodontal abscess, or tonsillitis. Regional lymphadenopathy, malaise, and low-grade fever are common. If edema or cellulitis extends to involve the masseter muscle, trismus often accompanies the condition. Pericoronitis is frequently complicated by pain induced by trauma from the opposing tooth during closure.

Pericoronitis is best managed by entering the follicular space, flushing the purulent material from the gingival sulcus with saline solution, and eliminating any occlusal trauma. Definitive treatment is usually extraction of the involved tooth. Antibiotic coverage is recommended when constitutional symptoms are present and the spread of infection is likely. Recurrences and chronicity are likely if the condition is managed only with antibiotics.

Periodontal Abscess (Figs. 9-5 and 9-6) A periodontal abscess is a fluctuant swelling of the gingiva resulting from pathogenic bacteria that are occluded in the gingival crevice. The condition is evidenced clinically by a smooth fluctuant nodule, increased mobility of the periodontally involved tooth, purulence, and tissue necrosis. Characteristically the attached gingiva is raised, red-purple, and without stippling or a free marginal groove. Patients often complain of well-localized, dull, and continuous pain, especially if the purulent exudate has no avenue for escape. Intensification of pain occurs when vertical or horizontal pressure is applied, or when the overlying soft tissue is palpated. Diagnostic evaluation utilizing a periodontal probe may initially produce discomfort, but is often therapeutic for a short time because it may drain the abscess. An unpleasant taste often accompanies the condition.

The pulp of a tooth associated with a periodontal abscess usually tests vital, unless the inflammatory process has extended into the pulp via the apex or accessory canals. Fever, malaise, and lymphadenopathy may coexist, and radiographic evidence of localized bone loss may be seen. Treatment should be directed toward necrotic material removal, adequate drainage, localized periodontal therapy, and improved plaque control measures. Failure to fully treat the problem can result in recurrence or spread of infection along fascial planes.

Epulis Fissuratum (Irritation Hyperplasia) (Figs. 9-7 and 9-8) The epulis fissuratum is a reactive inflammatory fibrous hyperplasia caused by a chronic irritant, usually the flange area of an old, poorly fitting complete or partial denture. Initially the overextended denture margin produces an ulcer that heals incompletely because of repeated trauma. Hyperplastic healing results and a pink-red, fleshy exuberance of mature granulation tissue is produced. The hyperplastic lesion, located where the denture flange rests, is found most commonly in females. It is nonpainful, grows slowly on either side of the denture, and causes the patient little concern.

The epulis fissuratum in the early stages consists of a single fold of smooth soft tissue. As the swelling grows, a central cleft or multiple clefts become apparent, the boundaries of which may drape over the denture flange. The mucolabial fold of the anterior region of the maxilla is the most common location, followed by the mandibular alveolar ridge and the mandibular lingual sulcus. Adjustment of the denture or construction of a new denture may reduce the trauma and inflammation, but will not cause the underlying fibrous tissue to regress. Likewise, surgical excision without alteration of the dentures promotes recurrence. Successful treatment usually requires surgical removal of the redundant tissue, microscopic examination of the excised tissue, and correction or reconstruction of the denture.

LOCALIZED GINGIVAL LESIONS

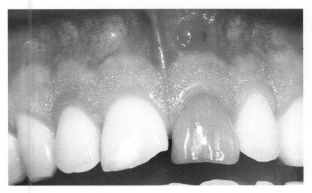

Fig. 9-1. Reddish **parulis** and discolored non-vital maxillary central incisor.

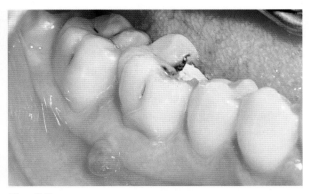

Fig. 9-2. Pink **parulis** at mucogingival junction adjacent to a non-vital first molar.

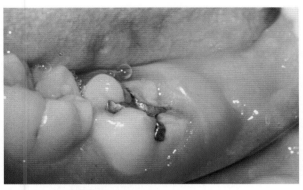

Fig. 9-3. Pericoronitis surrounding a partially erupted mandibular molar.

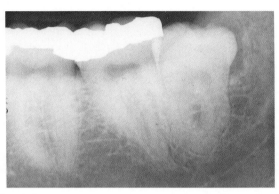

Fig. 9-4. Flame-shaped radiolucency of **pericoronitis** and underlying osteitis.

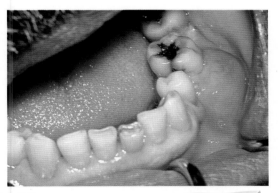

Fig. 9-5. Fluctuant swelling caused by a **periodontal abscess.**

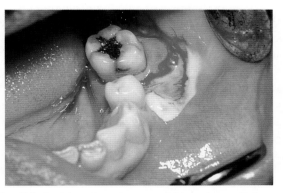

Fig. 9-6. Draining of purulent material from the **periodontal abscess** evident in Fig. 9-5.

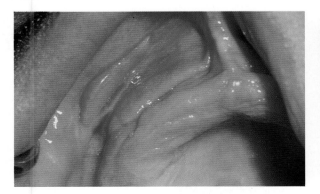

Fig. 9-7. Hyperplastic folds of an **epulis fissuratum** caused by irritation from a denture flange.

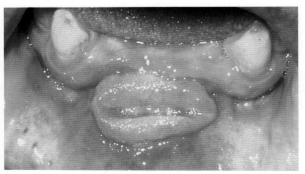

Fig. 9-8. Epulis fissuratum where the partial denture flange rests.

GENERALIZED GINGIVAL ENLARGEMENTS

Hereditary Fibromatosis Gingivae (Figs. 10-1 and 10-2) Hereditary fibromatosis gingivae is a rare progressive fibrous enlargement of the gingiva that is inherited as an autosomal dominant trait. The condition has an early childhood onset and becomes more prominent with age. The enlargement is usually generalized and noninflammatory, affecting the buccal and lingual surfaces of both jaws equally. The free, interproximal, and marginal gingiva are enlarged, uniformly pink in color, firm, nonhemorrhagic, and often nodular.

There are two varieties of hereditary fibromatosis gingivae: generalized and localized. The generalized type is nodular and diffuse, exhibiting multiple coalesced areas of globular gingival overgrowths that encroach on and eventually cover the crowns of the teeth. The localized variety is occasionally seen in which solitary overgrowths are limited to the palatal vault of the maxillary tuberosity or the lingual gingiva of the mandibular arch. These gingival overgrowths appear smooth, firm, and symmetrically round. The localized involvement may be unilateral or bilateral, and the term "focal gingival fibromatosis" has been suggested for this variant.

Hereditary fibromatosis gingivae may interfere with tooth eruption, mastication, and oral hygiene. In severe cases, noneruption of the primary or permanent teeth may be the chief complaint of the patient. Regression is not a feature of this disease, even with effective oral hygiene measures. Gingivectomy, with either a blade or a carbon dioxide laser, is the treatment of choice. Continued growth may require multiple operations. The condition may be accompanied by acromegalic facial features, hypertrichosis, or mental deficits.

Drug-Induced Gingival Hyperplasia (Figs. 10-3 and 10-4) In approximately 25 to 50% of patients taking the therapeutic prescription drugs phenytoin (Dilantin), nifedipine (Procardia), and cyclosporin-A, bulbous enlargement of the gingiva is a common side effect. The condition is usually seen in young patients after puberty, and can occur in either sex. Though the enlargement results from a hyperplastic response, an inflammatory component induced by dental bacterial plaque often coexists and tends to exacerbate the condition. The gingival enlargement is usually generalized and often appears most exaggerated on the labial aspects of the anterior teeth.

The overgrowth begins at the interdental papillae and enlarges to form soft red lumpy nodules that bleed easily. Progressive growth results in fibrotic changes: the interdental tissue becomes enlarged, pink, firm, and resilient to palpation. With time the condition can completely engulf the crowns of the teeth, which aggravates home care, limits mastication, and compromises aesthetics. Treatment may involve changing drug therapy and/or minimizing the overgrowth with meticulous plaque control measures. The gingival swelling usually does not completely regress even with reduced drug doses; thus, once present, the excess tissue often requires surgical removal.

Mouthbreathing (Figs. 10-5 and 10-6) Chronic mouthbreathing is characterized by nasal obstruction, a high narrow palatal vault, snoring, xerostomia, a sore throat upon wakening, and a characteristic form of gingivitis. Classically the gingival changes are limited to the anterior labial gingiva of the maxilla and, sometimes, the mandibular gingiva. These changes may be an incidental finding, or may be noticed in conjunction with caries limited to the incisors. Therefore, multiple anterior restorations often serve as a diagnostic clue.

Early changes involve diffuse redness of the labial, marginal and interdental gingiva. Shortly thereafter, the interproximal papillae become red, bulbous, and hemorrhagic. Progression of the condition results in inflammatory changes of the entire attached gingiva and bleeding upon probing. Improved oral hygiene will reduce the features, but will not resolve the condition.

The diagnosis of mouthbreathing is made by objective and subjective information. Confirmation is achieved when healing occurs after a protective dressing is placed on the affected gingiva at night, together with the return of gingivitis upon discontinuance of the dressings. Treatment should address the re-establishment of a patent nasal airway; thus, the aid of an otorhinolaryngologist is often required to effectively manage this condition.

Gingival Edema of Hypothyroidism (Figs. 10-7 and 10-8) Hypothyroidism is a relatively common disorder in which clinical manifestations are dependent on the age of onset, duration, and severity of the thyroid insufficiency. When the patient is deficient in hormone at an early age, cretinism results. This disease is characterized by short stature, mental retardation, disproportionate head-to-body size, delayed tooth eruption, mandibular micrognathism, and swollen lips and tongue. Regardless of the age of onset, hypothyroid patients exhibit coarse, dry, yellowish skin, intolerance to cold, and lethargy. Swelling is the classic feature and is most prominent in the face, particularly around the eyes.

Intraorally macroglossia and macrocheilia are common and may cause an altered speech pattern. The gingiva appears uniformly enlarged, pale pink in color, and compressible. Swelling occurs in all directions on both the facial and lingual sides of the dental arches. When secondary inflammation is present, the tissues become red and boggy and have a tendency to bleed easily. Treatment for the gingival condition depends on the degree of thyroid deficiency. Patients marginally deficient require only strict oral hygiene measures, whereas frank cases require supplemental thyroid therapy to achieve resolution of the systemic and oral condition.

GENERALIZED GINGIVAL ENLARGEMENTS

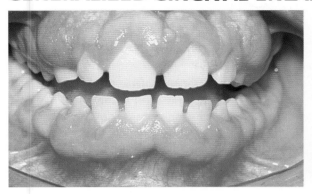

Fig. 10-1. Generalized gingival enlargement of **hereditary fibromatosis gingivae.** (Courtesy Dr Kenneth Abramovitch)

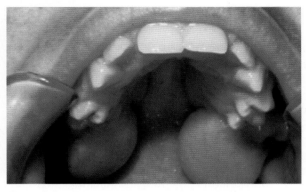

Fig. 10-2. Fibromatosis gingivae, localized type, limited to the tuberosity. (Courtesy Dr Ron Jorgenson)

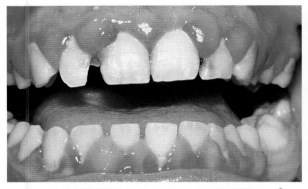

Fig. 10-3. Dilantin-induced gingival hyperplasia. (Courtesy Dr James Cottone)

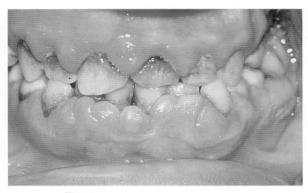

Fig. 10-4. Fibrotic **gingival hyperplasia** indicative of prolonged **dilantin therapy**.

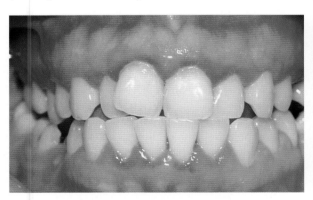

Fig. 10-5. Early gingival inflammation associated with **mouthbreathing.**

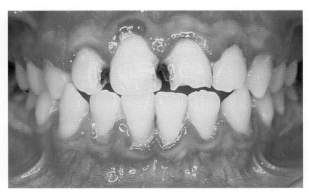

Fig. 10-6. Progressive gingival changes and caries seen in a chronic **mouthbreather.** (Courtesy Dr Charles Morris)

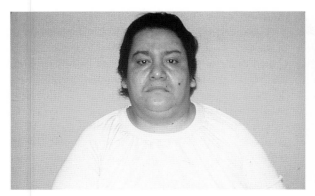

Fig. 10-7. A woman with **hypothyroidism** (myxedema).

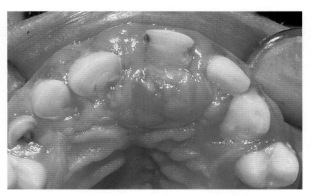

Fig. 10-8. Generalized gingival edema of **hypothyroidism;** same patient as in Fig. 10-7.

25

GINGIVITIS

Gingivitis (Figs. 11-1 and 11-2) Inflammation of the gingiva, or gingivitis, is the result of bacterial infection. Initially, gram-positive streptococcal organisms predominate. Over a 3-week period, however, gram-positive rods species, specifically *Actinomyces,* gram-negative organisms such as *Fusobacterium, Veillonella,* and spirochetal organisms including *Treponema* colonize the gingival sulcus. Persistence of supragingival microbial plaque results in characteristic gingival changes and the eventual establishment of subgingival microbial populations that may lead to periodontitis. Gingivitis can occur at any age, but most frequently arises during adolescence. It has no sexual or racial predilection.

Gingivitis can be classified according to distribution, duration, etiology, pathogenesis, and severity. The distribution may be general, local, marginal, or papillary; the duration acute or chronic. An abbreviated list of the different types of gingivitis based on etiology includes: actinomycotic, diabetic, hormonal, leukemic, plasma cell, psoriasiform, scorbutic, and human immunodeficiency virus (HIV).

Gingivitis is most often chronic and nonpainful, but acute, painful episodes may superimpose over the chronic state. The severity is often judged by the alterations in color, contour, and consistency, and by the presence of bleeding. Chronic gingivitis features red swollen marginal gingiva with bulbous interdental papillae that have a red-purple tinge. Stippling is lost as the marginal tissues enlarge. The condition may be difficult for the patient to control because hemorrhage and pain are induced by the slightest provocation; therefore patients will reduce brushing frequency and effectiveness. Treatment for acute and chronic forms of gingivitis consists of removal of dental plaque followed by daily oral hygiene measures.

Acute Necrotizing Ulcerative Gingivitis (Fig. 11-3)

A type of acute gingivitis that is linked to specific bacterial species and stress is termed "acute necrotizing ulcerative gingivitis" (ANUG), also known as Vincent's infection, or "trench mouth." This multifactorial disease has a bacterial population high in fusiform bacillae and spirochetes that can be demonstrated in smears using darkfield microscopy.

ANUG is characterized by fever, lymphadenopathy, malaise, fiery red gingiva, extreme oral pain, hypersalivation, and an unmistakable fetor oris. The interdental papillae are punched out, ulcerated and covered with a grayish pseudomembrane. ANUG is common in persons between the ages of 15 and 25, particularly students and military recruits enduring times of increased stress and reduced host resistance, and in patients with HIV infection. In rare instances the condition can extend onto other oral mucosal surfaces, or recur if mismanaged. Treatment of ANUG requires irrigation, gentle debridement, antibiotics (if constitutional symptoms are present), and stress reduction.

Partial loss of the interdental papillae can be expected despite normal healing.

Actinomycotic Gingivitis (Fig. 11-4) Actinomycotic gingivitis is a rare intraoral finding that may appear as a form of marginal gingivitis. Redness, intense burning pain, and lack of a response to normal therapeutic regimens are common features. A tissue biopsy reveals the non-acid fast, filamentous fungal organism. Gingivectomy or long-term antibiotic therapy provides effective treatment.

Hormonal Gingivitis (Pregnancy Gingivitis) (Figs. 11-5 and 11-6) Hormonal gingivitis is an inflammatory hyperplastic reaction to microbial plaque that generally affects females during puberty, pregnancy, or menopause. Although alteration in estrogen/progesterone levels as a result of hormonal shifts and the use of birth control pills have been implicated, the exact causative mechanism remains unknown.

The condition begins at the marginal and interdental gingiva and becomes most prominent interproximally. The marginal gingiva appears fiery red, swollen, and tender, while the papillae become compressible, swollen, and lumpy. Close inspection reveals hyperemic engorgement of the inflamed tissue. Severity is related to microbial accumulation; thus poor oral hygiene can exacerbate the condition, which is often the case with the gravid female, since tooth brushing may precipitate nausea. Hormonal gingivitis is usually transitory and responds to meticulous home care and frequent oral prophylaxis.

Diabetic Gingivitis (Figs. 11-7 and 11-8) Diabetes mellitus is a common disease affecting approximately 1 to 3% of the population in the United States. It is a progressive metabolic disorder characterized by hyperglycemia, glucosuria, polyuria, polydipsia, pruritis, and weight loss. Poor control of blood glucose levels is related to lack of production or utilization of insulin. Complications of diabetes include a variety of vascular-related problems such as atherosclerosis, retinopathy, peripheral forms of neuropathy, and renal failure. In addition, altered neutrophil chemotaxis increases the diabetic's risk of infection. A dry mouth, burning tongue, persistent gingivitis, or candidal infection may be the first intraoral signs of the disease.

The severity of diabetic gingivitis depends on the stage of the disease and the patient's oral hygiene. In the uncontrolled diabetic peculiar proliferations of exuberant tissue arise from the marginal and attached gingiva. The well-demarcated swellings are soft, red, irregular, and hemorrhagic. The surface of the hyperplastic tissue is usually bulbous and, in some cases, papulonodular. This type of gingivitis is difficult to manage when blood glucose levels remain elevated. Successful treatment requires meticulous home care and control of the blood glucose concentration with diet, hypoglycemic agents, or insulin.

GINGIVITIS

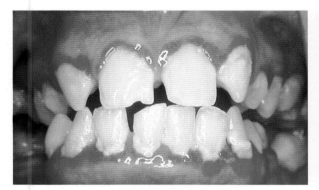
Fig. 11-1. Plaque-induced **marginal gingivitis.**

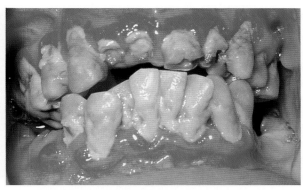
Fig. 11-2. Chronic gingivitis extending onto the attached gingiva. (Courtesy Dr Tom McDavid)

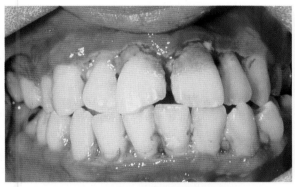
Fig. 11-3. Cratered papillae; **acute necrotizing ulcerative gingivitis** (ANUG). (Courtesy Dr Bill Baker)

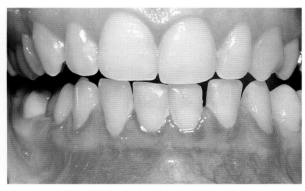
Fig. 11-4. Red, inflamed mandibular gingiva caused by Actinomyces infection of gingiva.

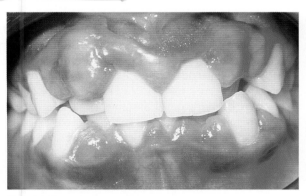
Fig. 11-5. Hormonal gingivitis in a pubertal female.

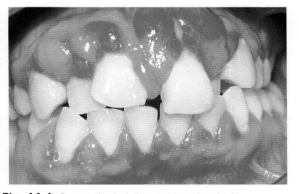
Fig. 11-6. Severe gingival changes associated with pregnancy; **hormonal ginigivitis.**

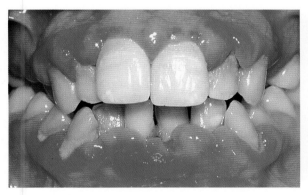
Fig. 11-7. Gingivitis in a 19-year-old woman with uncontrolled **diabetes mellitus.**

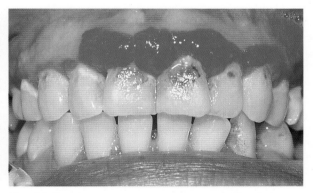
Fig. 11-8. Inflamed, papulonodular **hyperplasia of the gingiva** in a **diabetic patient.** (Courtesy Dr Margot Van Dis).

SPONTANEOUS GINGIVAL BLEEDING

Leukemic Gingivitis (Figs. 12-1 and 12-2)
Leukemia, a malignant condition characterized by white blood cell overproduction, is classified according to cell morphology (monocytic, myelogenous, or lymphoblastic) and the clinical course of the disease (acute or chronic). Oral manifestations are more frequently encountered in acute leukemia of the monocytic and myelogenous subtypes. Oral features occur early in the course of the disease because of neoplastic proliferation of one blood cell type, which reduces the normal production of the other hematopoietic cells.

Consistent signs of acute leukemia are cervical lymphadenopathy, malaise, anemic pallor, leukopenia-induced ulcerations, and gingival changes. Leukemic gingival tissues are usually red, tender, and spongy, and tend to peel away from the teeth. With progression of the disease the swollen gingiva becomes purple and shiny. Stippling of the tissue is lost and spontaneous bleeding from the gingival sulcus eventually occurs. The edematous tissue is most prominent interdentally and results from leukemic infiltration of white blood cells. In certain patients the neoplastic cells may invade pulpal and osseous tissue, inducing vague symptoms of pain without corresponding radiographic evidence of pathosis. Purpuric features such as petechial lesions and ecchymoses on pale mucosal membranes, together with gingival hemorrhage, occur frequently. Systemic control of leukemia often involves intensive radiotherapy, chemotherapy, blood transfusions, and bone marrow transplantation. Difficulty may be encountered in maintaining optimal oral health because of the chemotherapeutic-induced oral ulcerations. Meticulous oral hygiene combined with antimicrobial rinses is recommended to reduce the inflammatory and ulcerative sequelae of chemotherapy.

Agranulocytosis (Neutropenia) and Cyclic Neutropenia (Figs. 12-3 and 12-4) Neutropenia refers to a disease characterized by a decrease in the number of circulating polymorphonuclear neutrophils (PMNs). In most instances, the condition is recognized by its clinical symptoms, which consist of chronic infections and an almost complete absence of neutrophils in laboratory blood tests. Anti-metabolic, antibiotic, and cytotoxic drugs are the etiologic agents involved in over half of all cases. In rare instances the condition may be congenital. An uncontrollable infection in the neutropenic patient can result in bacterial pneumonia, sepsis, or death.

A distinct form of agranulocytosis is cyclic neutropenia, which is characterized by a periodic diminution of circulating PMNs that occurs about every 3 weeks and lasts for about 5 days. The condition is idiopathic and usually begins in childhood. It is sometimes accompanied by arthritis, pharyngitis, fever, headache, and lymphadenopa-

thy. A history of repeated infections of the ear and upper respiratory tract is common.

Intraorally patients demonstrate inflammatory gingival changes and mucosal ulcerations. The ulcerations are usually large, oval, and persistent. They vary in size and location; sometimes found on the attached gingiva and other times on the tongue and buccal mucosa. The gingivitis is periodic and ulcerative. At stages corresponding to elevated levels of PMNs, minimal inflammation is evident. In contrast, when the level of PMNs drops precipitously, generalized inflammatory hyperplasia and erythema occurs. If left untreated the condition is exacerbated by the presence of local factors such as plaque and calculus, resulting in alveolar bone loss, tooth mobility, and early exfoliation of teeth.

The periodic appearance and spontaneous regression of signs and symptoms should cause the clinician to suspect cyclic neutropenia. Daily repetition of the white blood cell count is required to diagnose this condition. Curative treatment is unavailable; therefore management is palliative, with antibiotic and antimicrobial therapy together with repeated oral prophylaxis.

Thrombocytopenic and Thrombocytopathic Purpura (Figs. 12-5 through 12-8) Platelets play an integral role in maintaining hemostasis by providing the primary hemostatic plug and by activating the intrinsic system of coagulation. A decrease in the number of circulating platelets (thrombocytopenia) may be idiopathic, or it may be due to decreased platelet production in the bone marrow, increased peripheral destruction, or increased splenic sequestration. Decreased function of circulating platelets (thrombocytopathia) is often related to hereditary syndromes or acquired states such as drug-induced bone marrow suppression, liver disease, or dysproteinemic states like uremia.

Vascular-related clinical manifestations of platelet disorders include petechiae, ecchymoses, epistaxis, hematuria, hypermenorrhea, and gastrointestinal bleeding resulting in melena. Spontaneous gingival bleeding is a frequent, early, and dramatic occurrence. The blood oozes from the gingival sulcus profusely, either spontaneously or following minor trauma such as toothbrushing. Later the fluid turns into purplish-black globs of clotted blood that adhere to the oral structures. Occasionally, clotted blood may be swallowed, which results in nausea. Mild traumas, particularly at the occlusal line of the buccal mucosa and tongue, are sites of extensive hemorrhage. Multifocal red petechial spots on the soft palate is another frequent clinical sign of bleeding disorders. The platelet count, clot retraction time, tourniquet test, and template bleeding time should be ordered to diagnose a platelet disorder. Platelet transfusions may be necessary if local measures prove ineffective in controlling oral bleeding.

SPONTANEOUS GINGIVAL BLEEDING

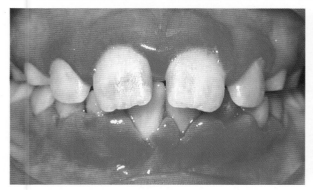

Fig. 12-1. Swollen, shiny, bleeding gingiva of a patient with **acute myelogenous leukemia.** (Courtesy Dr Monique Michaud)

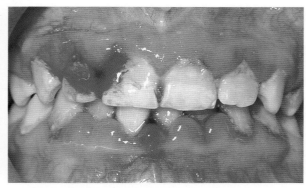

Fig. 12-2. **Acute lymphocytic leukemia;** gingival enlargement and spontaneous bleeding. (Courtesy Dr Monique Michaud)

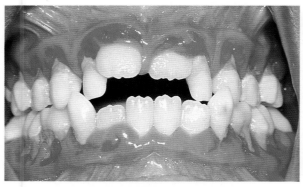

Fig. 12-3. **Cyclic neutropenia** associated gingival erythema and epithelial erosion.

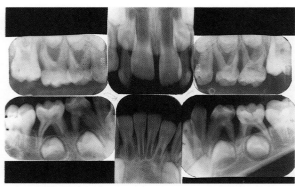

Fig. 12-4. Radiograph revealing loss of periodontal support and floating teeth; same patient with **cyclic neutropenia** as in Fig. 12-3.

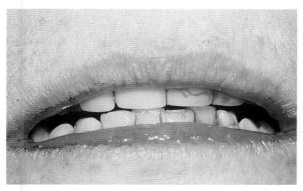

Fig. 12-5. Patient with **cirrhosis** of the liver and a **clotting-factor deficiency.** (Courtesy Dr Roger Rao)

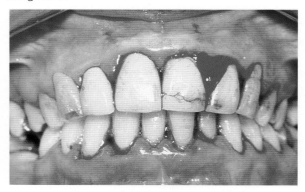

Fig. 12-6. **Spontaneous gingival bleeding** of same patient with **cirrhosis** in Fig. 12-5. (Courtesy Dr Roger Rao)

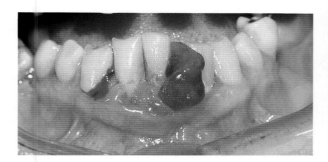

Fig. 12-7. **Thrombocytopenia;** gingival bleeding and the resultant blood clot. (Courtesy Dr Larry Skoczylas)

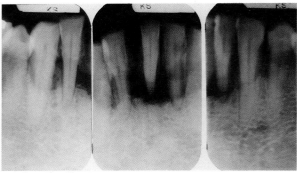

Fig. 12-8. Radiographic evidence of chronic irritants that caused the bleeding seen in patient with **thrombocytopenia** in Fig. 12-7.

SWELLINGS OF THE LIP

Angioedema (Angioneurotic Edema) (Figs. 13-1 and 13-2) Angioedema is a hypersensitivity reaction characterized by the accumulation of fluid within the facial tissues, resulting in soft, swollen areas under the skin. It occurs in hereditary and acquired forms, and may be generalized or localized. When the nonpainful swelling affects the lips it is usually uniform and diffuse, but may be asymmetrical, involving parts of the lip in varying degrees. Angioedema develops within minutes or gradually over a few hours, and is of transient duration. The vermilion border appears stretched, everted, pliable, and less distinct than usual, whereas the surface epithelium remains normal in color, or is slightly red. Swellings of the tongue, floor of the mouth, eyelids, face, and extremities may accompany the condition, and complaints of burning or itching are common.

Although the cause of angioedema is poorly understood, foods, wine, drugs, and stressful situations may be causative factors for the acquired type. In this form of the disease, antigenic stimuli appear to trigger an immunoglobulin-linked, histamine-mediated increase in capillary permeability. The hereditary type, on the other hand, appears to be linked to an enzyme deficiency.

Angioneurotic edema is usually recurrent and self-limiting. Generally it poses little threat to the patient. Withdrawal of the allergen together with the administration of antihistamines is the treatment of choice. In cases involving swelling of the pharyngeal tissues, airway compromise is of prime concern.

Cheilitis Glandularis (Fig. 13-3) Cheilitis glandularis is of unknown etiology and is most frequently encountered in adult males. It is a chronic inflammatory disorder of the accessory labial salivary glands, particularly those of the lower lip, that is characterized by diffuse enlargement and eversion of the lip. Although poorly understood, this condition may be associated with smoking, poor oral hygiene, or chronic exposure to the sun and wind; it may also be attributable to bacterial infection or congenital disposition.

Cheilitis glandularis clinically produces a symmetrically enlarged, everted, and firm lower lip. As time passes, the inflamed labial accessory salivary glands become dilated and appear as multiple small red spots. From these ductal openings a viscous, yellowish, mucopurulent exudate is secreted that can cover the entire lip, making it sticky. Progression of the condition causes the lip to appear atrophic, dry, fissured, and scaly. Distinction of the vermilion border is eventually lost, and secondary infection of a deep labial fissure often results in fistulation and scarring. Emollients and sunscreens afford protection, but severe cases require vermilionectomy, which produces an excellent esthetic result. Patients with cheilitis glandularis are at an increased risk of malignant transformation.

Cheilitis Granulomatosa (Figs. 13-4 through 13-6) Cheilitis granulomatosa is a noncaseating granulomatous condition resulting in nonpainful symmetric enlargement of the lips. Its etiology is unknown, and it has no sexual predilection. The swelling, which involves the entire lip, is large and develops slowly at a young age. Both lips may be firm and swollen, but symmetric enlargement of the lower lip is more common. The diffuse enlargement is asymptomatic and does not affect the color of the lip, but discrete nodules can often be palpated. Granulomatous swellings of the tongue, buccal mucosa, gingiva, palatal mucosa, and face have also been associated with this condition. When unilateral facial paralysis and a fissured pebbly tongue are exhibited, the Melkersson-Rosenthal syndrome should be suspected. Steroids and surgery have been used with limited success, while in selected patients elimination of an odontogenic infection has proved curative. Spontaneous regression is possible.

Trauma (Fig. 13-7) Trauma to the lips often results in edema that is fluctuant, irregular, and exquisitely painful. The trauma may originate from an external source or it may be self-induced. External trauma may damage the soft tissue of the lip, resulting in laceration or hemorrhage. Tooth fracture may accompany the condition.

Traumatic enlargement of the lip is often a problem of children and mentally handicapped patients who inadvertently chew their lip while under local anesthesia. The best management for this type of lip injury is to limit the traumatic influence, apply ice compresses, and treat any lacerations or hemorrhage as soon as possible.

Cellulitis (Fig. 13-8) Cellulitis, in the strictest sense, means "inflammation of the cellular tissue." This degenerative process is caused by a bacterial infection in which localization of purulent material has yet to occur. When of dental origin, it typically produces grossly edematous facial tissue that is warm and painful to touch and is extremely hard to palpation.

A firm, diffusely swollen lip may be the first sign of cellulitis of odontogenic origin. A nonvital tooth is usually the root of the problem, and is where the bacterial invasion begins. Failure of host defense mechanisms to control the infection usually results in inflammatory edema, pus formation, and a clinically evident swelling of the vestibule, cheek, and/or lip. Delay in initiating treatment can result in cervical lymphadenopathy, malaise, trismus, encroachment of the swelling on the lower eyelid, elevated temperature, and increased pulse. Treatment involves extirpation of necrotic pulpal tissue, drainage, culture, antibiotic sensitivity testing, and antibiotic therapy. Injection of local anesthetic into the inflammatory region should be avoided to minimize spread of the infection.

30

SWELLINGS OF THE LIP

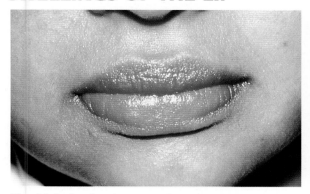

Fig. 13-1. Swollen lower lip of **angioedema.** (Courtesy Dr Linda Otis)

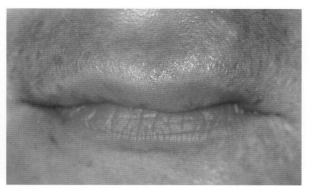

Fig. 13-2. Reddish, edematous upper lip and philtrum indicative of **angioedema.**

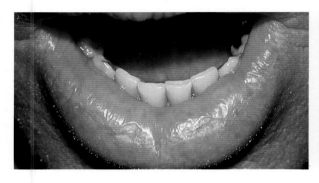

Fig. 13-3. Enlarged, everted lower lip with discrete red spots of **cheilitis glandularis.**

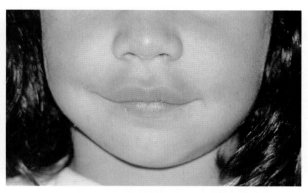

Fig. 13-4. Melkerson-Rosenthal syndrome, cheilitis granulomatosa, and facial paralysis.

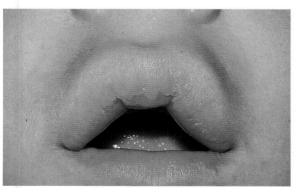

Fig. 13-5. Symmetric enlargement of the upper lip; same patient with **Melkerson-Rosenthal syndrome** as in Fig. 13-4.

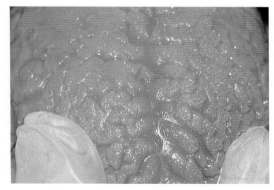

Fig. 13-6. Fissured tongue; same patient with **Melkerson-Rosenthal syndrome** as in Fig. 13-4.

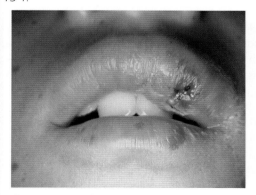

Fig. 13-7. Traumatic swelling of the upper lip.

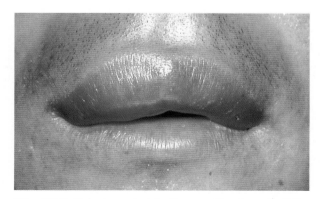

Fig. 13-8. Odontogenic infection resulting in **cellulitis** and a swollen upper lip. (Courtesy Dr Geza Terezhalmy)

NODULES OF THE LIP

Mucocele (Mucous Retention Phenomenon, Mucous Retention Cyst) (Figs. 14-1 and 14-2)

The retention of mucous secretions in subepithelial tissue is called a mucous retention phenomenon, which has been subdivided into two types. The first type, the mucous retention phenomenon-retention type, or mucous retention cyst, is lined by ductal epithelium and results from the pooling of mucous in an obstructed and dilated excretory duct. The second type, the mucous retention phenomenon-extravasation type, or mucous extravasation cyst, lacks an epithelial lining. It is usually surrounded by granulomatous tissue and results from traumatic severing of a duct followed by the subsequent pooling of mucous outside of the accessory salivary gland duct in the connective tissue.

The mucous retention phenomenon constitutes the most common nodular swelling of the lower lip and, as such, is specifically termed the mucocele. These swellings are asymptomatic, soft, fluctuant, bluish-gray, and usually less than 1 cm in diameter. Enlargement coincident with meals may be an occasional finding. The most common location is the lower lip midway between the midline and commissure, but other locations include the buccal mucosa, palate, floor of the mouth, and ventral tongue. Children and young adults are most frequently affected. Trauma is the etiologic agent, which predisposes the lesions to recurrence. Patients usually have esthetic concerns and desire surgical removal of the lesion. The lesion is negative to diascopy, but yields a semi-clear fluid upon aspiration. Treatment is excisional biopsy and histopathologic examination. Recurrence, though rare, is possible if the mucocele is not properly excised or if other ducts are severed during surgery.

Accessory Salivary Gland Tumor (Figs. 14-3 and 14-4)

Nodular swellings of the upper lip are infrequent and are usually caused by benign neoplasia of the minor salivary glands, i.e., the canalicular or monomorphic adenoma, and the pleomorphic adenoma. Benign accessory salivary gland tumors constitute approximately 10% of all salivary gland tumors and are characterized by encapsulation, slow growth, and long duration (several months). Persons over the age of 30 are usually affected. Clinically the pleomorphic adenoma is a pink to purple dome-shaped or multinodular lesion that commonly protrudes from the inner aspect of the lip or vestibule. It is usually semi-solid, freely movable, painless, and especially firm on palpation. The border is well-circumscribed, and although it has unlimited potential for growth, the tumor generally remains less than 2 cm in diameter. Fluctuance and surface ulceration are not usual clinical features.

Malignant salivary gland tumors are rare in the upper lip and may be distinguished from benign neoplasia by their rapid and aggressive growth, short duration, and tendency to ulcerate and cause neurologic symptoms. Treatment for salivary gland neoplasia consists of surgical excision. If the excision is incomplete, recurrences are possible.

Nasolabial Cyst (Nasoalveolar Cyst) (Figs. 14-5 and 14-6)

The nasolabial cyst, or nasoalveolar cyst, is a fissural cyst of soft tissue located intraorally in the cuspid-lateral incisor portion of the upper lip. The etiology is uncertain, and two theories have been suggested. The most accepted theory is that epithelial remnants become entrapped during the embryologic fusion of the lateral nasal, globular, and maxillary processes. A more recent theory suggests that the tissue originates from the nasolacrimal duct. Proliferation and cystic degeneration of the entrapped tissue usually do not become clinically evident until after age 30, even though the tissue has been entrapped since birth. The condition has a slight female predilection.

The nasolabial cyst is a palpable soft tissue mass under the upper lip that may cause elevation of the ala of the nose, as well as dilation of the nostril and alteration of the nasolabial fold. The cyst may be tense or fluctuant, depending on size. Aspiration will yield a yellowish or straw-colored fluid. It is most often unilateral and is generally not in contact with the adjacent bone; thus the maxillary teeth remain vital. Infrequently, if the nasolabial cyst applies pressure to the adjacent bone, local resorption of osseous structures can result. Treatment is simple excision.

Implantation Cyst (Epithelial Inclusion Cyst) (Fig. 14-7)

An implantation cyst is an unusual cyst arising from a foreign-body reaction to surface epithelium that is implanted within epidermal structures after traumatic laceration. The cyst can occur intraorally or extraorally, at any age, and in any race or sex. Within the mouth the lesion appears as a firm, dome-shaped, freely movable nodule located at the site of impetus, which is often the lip. Implantation cysts are usually small, solitary, and asymptomatic. Growth appears to remain constant, and the overlying mucosa appears smooth and pink. A previous history of trauma should lead the clinician to suspect this lesion. Surgical excision and histopathologic examination is recommended.

Mesenchymal Tumors (Fig. 14-8)

A variety of mesenchymal tumors can cause nodular swellings of the lip. One example is the neurofibroma. Neurofibromas may be solitary or found in conjunction with von Recklinghausen's disease. When solitary, the neurofibroma is usually an asymptomatic, sessile, smooth-surfaced nodule of the buccal mucosa, gingiva, palate, or lips. Histologically the tumor consists of connective tissue and nerve fibrils. The discovery of a solitary neurofibroma requires close examination for multiple neurofibromatosis, since the latter condition is associated with a marked tendency toward malignant transformation.

NODULES OF THE LIP

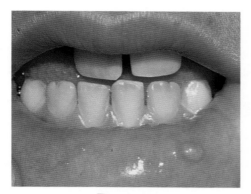

Fig. 14-1. Small bluish **mucocele** of the mandibular labial mucosa.

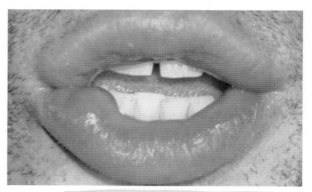

Fig. 14-2. Large dome-shaped **mucocele** that appeared following trauma.

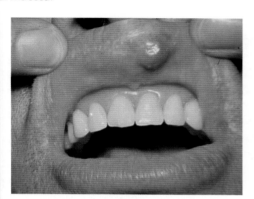

Fig. 14-3. Pleomorphic adenoma; a firm bluish nodule.

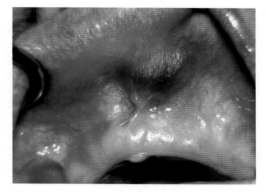

Fig. 14-4. Purplish **canalicular adenoma** of the maxillary labial mucosa.

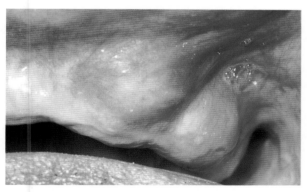

Fig. 14-5. Nasolabial cyst; a fluctuant nodule on palpation.

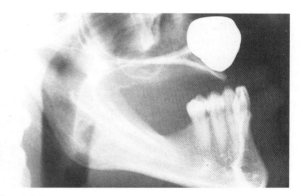

Fig. 14-6. Lateral skull radiograph of a **nasolabial cyst** injected with contrast medium. (Courtesy Dr Chris Nortjé)

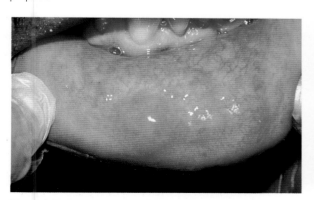

Fig. 14-7. Trauma-induced **implantation cyst.**

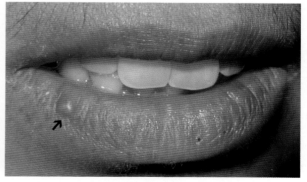

Fig. 14-8. Small **neurofibroma** of the lower lip. (Courtesy Dr John McDowell)

CONDITIONS PECULIAR TO THE LIP

Actinic Cheilitis (Solar Elastosis) (Figs. 15-1 and 15-2) Actinic cheilitis is a clinical lesion of the lower lip due to excessive solar radiation damage. Elderly fair-skinned men with outdoor occupations are typically affected. In early stages, the lower lip is mildly keratotic with a subtle blending of the vermilion border with the adjacent skin. With increased exposure to the sun, focal white zones that have distinct or diffuse borders become apparent. Slowly the lip becomes firm, scaly, slightly swollen, and everted. Ulceration with encrustation is typical of the chronic condition. Development of ulcerations may be due to loss of elasticity, or they may be an early sign of carcinomatous transformation. Histologic features include atrophic thinning of the epithelium, subepithelial basophilic degeneration of collagen, and increased elastin fibers. Biopsy is recommended to rule out other sun-related diseases that should be distinguished from actinic cheilitis, including epithelial dysplasia, carcinoma in situ, basal cell carcinoma, squamous cell carcinoma, malignant melanoma, keratoacanthoma, cheilitis glandularis, and herpes labialis.

Actinic cheilitis is considered a precancerous condition and should be treated accordingly. Clinicians should warn the patient of the likelihood of disease progression without the use of sunscreen protectives. Dysplastic changes should be treated surgically or by topical application of 5-fluorouracil.

Monilial Cheilitis (Figs. 15-3 and 15-4) Monilial cheilitis is an inflammatory condition of the lips associated with *Candida albicans* and a lip-licking habit. It is believed that the candidal organisms obtain access to the surface layers of the labial epithelium following mucosal breakdown, which is caused by repeated wetting and drying of the labial tissues. Desquamation of the surface epithelium results, and a fine whitish scale consisting of dried salivary mucous may be seen. In children the affected perilabial skin appears red, atrophic, and fissured. Chapped, dry, itchy, burning lips and the inability to eat hot spicy foods are frequent complaints. Chronic situations are characterized by painful vertical fissures that ulcerate and are slow to heal. A hypersensitivity reaction to ingredients contained within lip balms or lip sticks may mimic the condition. In monilial cheilitis the lip-licking habit perpetuates the condition. Although nystatin ointment is helpful, ultimate resolution requires habit elimination.

Angular Cheilitis (Perleche) (Figs. 15-5 and 15-6) Angular cheilitis is a painful condition consisting of radiating erythematous fissures at the corners of the mouth. The condition is most commonly seen after the age of 50 and is usually encountered in females and denture wearers. The etiology is believed to be associated with a mixed infection of *Candida albicans* and *Staphylococcus aureaus*.

The linear abrasions of angular cheilitis result from repeated pooling of saliva. Initially the mucocutaneous tissue at the corners of the mouth become soft, red, and ulcerated. With time the erythematous fissures become deep and extend several centimeters from the commissure onto the perilabial skin, or they ulcerate and involve the labial and buccal mucosa. The ulcers frequently develop crusts that split and reulcerate during normal oral function. Small yellow-brown granulomatous nodules may eventually appear. Bleeding is infrequent.

Angular cheilitis is chronic, usually bilateral, and often associated with denture stomatitis or glossitis. Predisposing conditions include anemia, poor oral hygiene, frequent use of broad-spectrum antibiotics, decreased vertical dimension, flaccid perioral folds, and vitamin B-group nutritional deficiency. Treatment should include preventive measures (such as elimination of traumatic factors, meticulous oral hygiene, and reestablishment of the correct vertical dimension) combined with topical antifungal and antibiotic therapy. Vitamin supplementation may also prove beneficial.

Exfoliative Cheilitis (Figs. 15-7 and 15-8) Exfoliative cheilitis is a persistent condition affecting the lips that is characterized by fissuring, desquamation, and the formation of hemorrhagic crusts. *Candida albicans*, oral sepsis, stress, and habitual lip biting are etiologic agents. This condition usually begins as a single fissure near the midline of the lower lip and spreads to produce multiple fissures. The fissures may ultimately develop a yellow-white scale or ulcerate and form hemorrhagic crusts over the entire lip. The condition is often bothersome and unsightly, with the lower lip being more adversely affected than the upper lip. When the condition is symptomatic, burning is the usual chief complaint. Exfoliative cheilitis has a predisposition for teenage girls and young women, and stress has been reported to cause acute exacerbations. Because the condition appears to be multifactorial, exfoliative cheilitis is difficult to manage and may persist for many years. Treatment is best rendered through the elimination of predisposing factors together with topical application of antifungal ointments.

CONDITIONS PECULIAR TO THE LIP

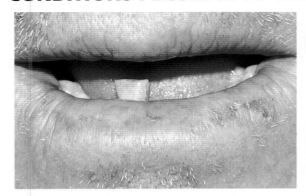

Fig. 15-1. Actinic cheilitis; loss of the vermilion border of lower lip, due to chronic sun exposure.

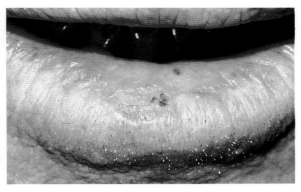

Fig. 15-2. Keratotic foci and thickened lower lip associated with **actinic cheilitis.**

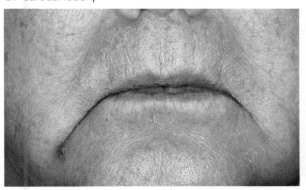

Fig. 15-3. Monilial cheilitis with characteristic whitish scale and red inflammatory borders. (Courtesy Dr Curt Lundeen)

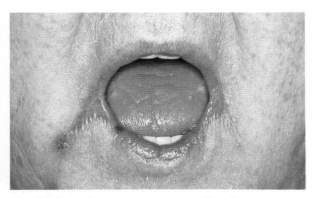

Fig. 15-4. Desquamation and fissuring of the lips caused by <u>Candida</u> infection; **monilial cheilitis.**

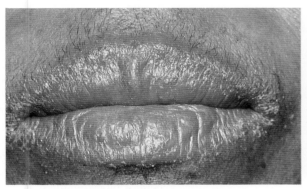

Fig. 15-5. Flabby perioral folds and **angular cheilitis.**

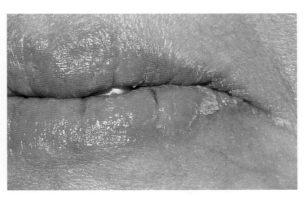

Fig. 15-6. Erythematous areas extending from the corners of mouth indicative of **angular cheilitis.**

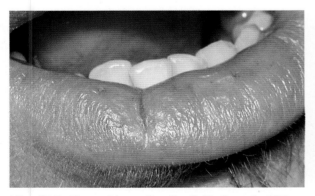

Fig. 15-7. Fissured lower lip of **exfoliative cheilitis.**

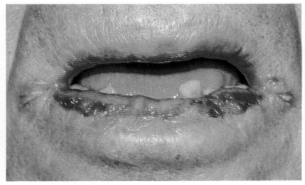

Fig. 15-8. Hemorrhagic crusts of a severe case of **exfoliative cheilitis.**

PALATAL SWELLINGS

Palatal Tori (Torus Palatinus) **(Figs. 16-1 and 16-2)** A palatal torus is a form of bony exostosis that affects approximately 20% of the adult population. It is frequently inherited; thus multiple family members are affected. The incidence of palatal tori is higher in females than it is in males.

Tori vary greatly in clinical size and shape, and they tend to increase slowly in all dimensions after puberty. The location is always in the midline of the hard palate adjacent to either the bicuspid or molar teeth. The torus palatinus is usually a single, smooth, dome-shaped, bony-hard swelling; however, bosselated versions are occasionally seen with a midline groove and several locular outgrowths. The covering mucosa is pale pink, thin, and delicate; the boundary of the lesion is delineated from the palatal vault by a raised oval contour.

The palatal torus is frequently asymptomatic unless traumatized, and patients may insist that they were unaware of the torus's presence until the traumatic episode occurs. The resultant ulcer should always be observed until resolution; if healing does not occur chronic irritants should be identified and eliminated. Palatal tori should be removed if they interfere with phonetics, mastication, or the construction of prosthetic appliances.

Incisive Canal Cyst (Nasopalatine Duct Cyst) **(Figs. 16-3 and 16-4)** The incisive canal cyst is a developmental cyst that forms from entrapped squamous or respiratory epithelial remnants. It may occur at any age and anywhere along the course of the incisive canal, but generally the cyst is confined to the palatal bone between the maxillary central incisors at the height of the incisive canal.

The incisive canal cyst is usually asymptomatic and is discovered as an incidental finding during routine examination. Symptomatic cysts are usually bacterially infected. Infrequently the cyst arises entirely in the soft tissue of the incisive papilla, where it appears as a small, superficial, fluctuant swelling. A well-developed incisive canal cyst may swell the entire anterior third of the hard palate.

The radiographic features of the incisive canal cyst are characteristic. The cyst appears as a well-delineated, midline, symmetrically oval or heart-shaped radiolucency located between the roots of vital maxillary central incisors. The cystic border is contiguous with the incisive canal and may vary greatly in size. Root divergence and root resorption of the central incisors are occasional findings associated with large cystic lesions. A similar cyst that is located more posteriorly in the palate has been referred to as the median palatal cyst. Current beliefs are that the incisive canal cyst and the median palatal cyst represent the same anomaly found in slightly different locations. Treatment for both is surgical enucleation.

Periapical Abscess (Figs. 16-5 and 16-6) A periapical abscess is a fluctuant soft-tissue swelling consisting of purulent material that results from bacterial infection of the pulp. It appears adjacent to a diseased tooth, which is often tender to percussion, mobile, and slightly "high" in occlusion. Regional lymphadenopathy, fever, malaise, and trismus are common accompanying features. Careful examination of the teeth and their supporting tissues along with diagnostic testing reveals the offending nonvital tooth. Radiographically an oval periapical radiolucency is usually seen.

Any abscessed maxillary tooth may produce a swelling of the palate. Generally the swelling is red-purple, soft, tender, and lateral to the midline if a maxillary posterior tooth is involved. In contrast, an abscessed maxillary incisor may cause a midline swelling in the anterior third of the palate. Aspiration or incision produces a creamy yellow or yellow-green purulent discharge. Immediate drainage, endodontic therapy, or extraction is indicated to prevent spread of the infection. Antibiotics, analgesics, and antipyretics may also be needed.

Benign Lymphoid Hyperplasia (Follicular Lymphoid Hyperplasia) (Figs. 16-7 and 16-8) Benign lymphoid hyperplasia is a rare, benign, reactive process that involves proliferation of the lymphoid tissue of the palate. Persons over the age of 50 are most commonly affected. The etiology is unknown. Authorities dispute whether the proliferation is a reaction to regional or generalized stimuli.

Clinically the exuberant lesion arises at the posterior extent of the hard palate and grows slowly, either unilaterally or bilaterally. The enlargement may reach 3 cm in diameter, yet patients rarely complain of pain. The surface of the mature lesion is pink to purple, nonulcerated, and dome-shaped or lumpy. The mass is usually soft, but on occasion may be firm to palpation. Surgical excision is the treatment of choice, followed by radiation therapy if the lesion recurs. The condition may clinically resemble palatal lymphoma, benign lymphoepithelial lesion, and Sjögren's syndrome, whereas histological features often mimic nodular lymphoma. Fortunately, benign lymphoid hyperplasia fails to disseminate like lymphoma.

PALATAL SWELLINGS

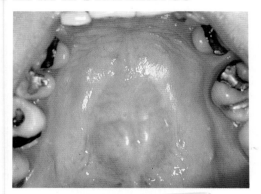

Fig. 16-1. Torus palatinus, slightly lobulated.

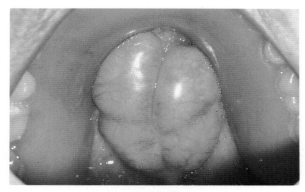

Fig. 16-2. Lobular **torus palatinus** with a denture situated around the torus.

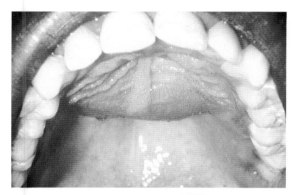

Fig. 16-3. Fluctuant **incisive canal cyst** involving the anterior third of the palate. (Courtesy Dr Geza Terezhalmy)

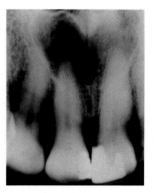

Fig. 16-4. Heart-shaped radiolucency characteristic of an **incisive canal cyst.** (Courtesy Dr Olaf Langland)

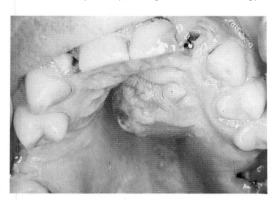

Fig. 16-5. Periapical abscess arising from the non-vital maxillary lateral incisor.

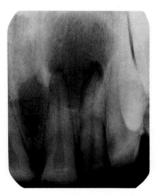

Fig. 16-6. Radiolucency typical of a **periapical abscess.**

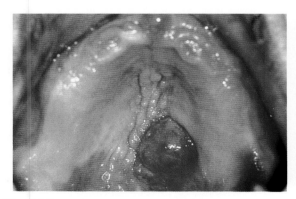

Fig. 16-7. Benign lymphoid hyperplasia arising at the junction of hard and soft palate. (Courtesy Dr Dale Miles)

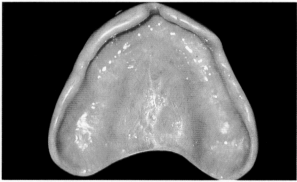

Fig. 16-8. Inappropriate management of **benign lymphoid hyperplasia**: denture accomodates nodule seen in Fig. 16-7. (Courtesy Dr Dale Miles)

PALATAL SWELLINGS

Necrotizing Sialometaplasia (Figs. 17-1 and 17-2)
Necrotizing sialometaplasia is a benign reactive lesion, chiefly of accessory palatal salivary glands, that has histologic features suggestive of malignancy. The inflammatory lesion begins after trauma as a rapidly growing nodular swelling on the lateral aspect of the hard palate, particularly of adult males. Tissue infarction as a result of vasoconstriction and ischemia has been implicated in the pathogenesis of this condition. Rarely the soft palate or buccal mucosa is involved, and bilateral cases have been reported.

Initially, necrotizing sialometaplasia is a small painless nodule that eventually enlarges and ulcerates, causing pain. The size of the soft tissue swelling is variable, and growth up to 2 cm is possible. A deep central ulcer with a grayish pseudomembrane is characteristic. The surface of the depressed ulcer is irregular and pebbly, and the border is often rolled. Healing occurs spontaneously over 4 to 8 weeks. Biopsy is recommended to rule out similar-appearing lesions such as salivary gland tumors and malignant lymphoma. Necrotizing sialometaplasia demonstrates squamous metaplasia of ductal epithelium, which may be misdiagnosed for mucoepidermoid carcinoma or adenocarcinoma of the palate.

Benign Accessory Salivary Gland Neoplasm (Figs. 17-3 and 17-4)
The pleomorphic adenoma, or benign mixed tumor, is the most common benign neoplasm of accessory salivary glands. It occurs in major or minor salivary glands, and the palate is the most common location when accessory salivary glands are affected. Occurrences are most frequent in females between the ages of 30 and 60. They tend to occur lateral to the midline and distal to the anterior third of the hard palate.

The classic clinical presentation of the pleomorphic adenoma is a firm painless, nonulcerated, irregularly dome-shaped swelling. Palpation may reveal isolated softer areas and a smooth or lobulated surface. Slow persistent enlargement over a period of years is typical, and lesions may achieve sizes greater than 1.5 cm in diameter. Histologically this tumor has epithelial cells in a nestlike arrangement, with pools of myxoid, chondroid, and mucoid material. A distinct fibrous connective tissue capsule containing tumor cells surrounds and usually limits the extension of the tumor. Thorough excisional biopsy is the recommended treatment, since recurrences are frequent following simple enucleation or incomplete excision. Tumorous involvement of the capsule may play a role in recurrence.

The monomorphic adenoma is a benign salivary gland tumor that can occur in the palate. It consists of a regular glandular pattern, usually one cell type, and lacks a mesenchymal component like that of the pleomorphic adenoma. Treatment is surgical excision.

Malignant Accessory Salivary Gland Neoplasm (Figs. 17-5 and 17-6)
Adenoid cystic carcinoma (cylindroma) and mucoepidermoid carcinoma are the two most common intraoral malignant accessory salivary gland neoplasms. Persons between the ages of 20 and 50 are most frequently affected by the mucoepidermoid tumor, whereas the adenoid cystic carcinoma usually occurs after the age of 50. In addition to salivary glands, adenoid cystic carcinoma occurs in respiratory, gastrointestinal, and reproductive tissues, whereas mucoepidermoid tumor may occur in the skin, respiratory tract, or centrally within bone, particularly the mandible.

Malignant accessory salivary gland neoplasms occur frequently in the posterior palate. Classically they are asymptomatic, firm, dome-shaped swellings that occur lateral to the midline. The overlying tissue appears normal in the early stages, but later the mucosa becomes erythematous, with multiple small telangieactactic surface vessels. Growth is more rapid and more painful than with benign salivary gland tumors. Induration and eventual spontaneous ulceration are common, indicating rapid malignant growth. A bluish appearance and/or a mucous exudate emanating from the ulcerated surface of the swelling are distinctive for mucoepidermoid carcinoma.

Treatment is usually radical excision. The prognosis varies depending upon the degree of histologic differentiation, the extent of the lesion, and the presence of metastasis. Adenoid cystic carcinoma rarely metastasizes but is an infiltrating malignancy with a propensity for distant spread by perineural invasion; therefore lifetime followup is necessary. In contrast, the mucoepidermoid tumor infrequently metastasizes and is more easily cured by surgical means.

Primary Lymphoma of the Palate (Figs. 17-7 and 17-8)
Malignant lymphomas are solid neoplastic growths of lymphocytes or histiocytes that are classified into Hodgkin's or non-Hodgkin's lymphoma and subdivided between nodal and extranodal disease. Primary non-Hodgkin's lymphoma may develop at any site at which lymphoid tissue is present, including the cervical lymph nodes, mandible, and palate. When the primary lesion affects the palate the condition is sometimes referred to as lymphoproliferative disease of the palate. Rarely lymphoma may affect the gingiva.

Primary lymphomas of the palate occur most commonly in patients over the age of 60, but may be seen in younger patients, especially those with AIDS. Primary lymphomas may be solitary or associated with widespread disease, though they usually precede disseminated disease. Clinically the lesion arises at the junction of the hard and soft palates. The slow-growing palatal swelling is asymptomatic, soft, spongy, and nonulcerated, and rarely affects the underlying palatal bone. The surface is often lumpy and pink to blue-purple in color. Early recognition and biopsy is extremely important, as the disease may be confined entirely to the palate in the early stages. Palatal lymphomas are usually irradiated, whereas disseminated disease necessitates the use of chemotherapy.

PALATAL SWELLINGS

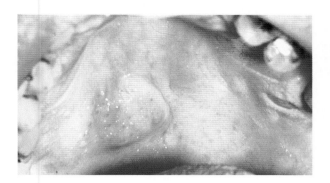

Fig. 17-1. Rapidly growing swelling of lateral hard palate; **necrotizing sialometaplasia.** (Courtesy Dr Dale Buller)

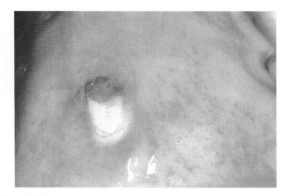

Fig. 17-2. One week later, **necrotizing sialometaplasia** appeared as a large depressed ulcer. (Courtesy Dr J. L. Jensen)

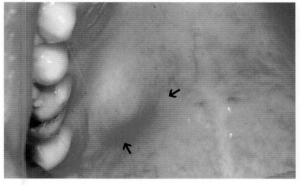

Fig. 17-3. Slow growing firm nodule; **pleomorphic adenoma.** (Courtesy Dr James Cottone)

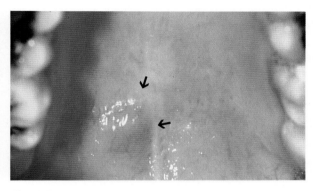

Fig. 17-4. Asymptomatic **monomorphic adenoma** in a 25-year-old female. (Courtesy Dr S. Brent Dove)

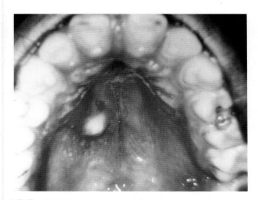

Fig. 17-5. Whitish mucous exuding from a **mucoepidermoid carcinoma.** (Courtesy Dr Jack Sherman)

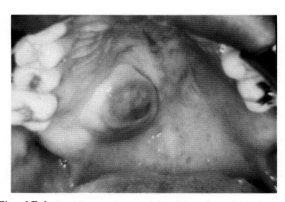

Fig. 17-6. Rapidly growing nodule with surface ulceration; **adenoid cystic carcinoma.**

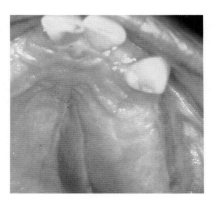

Fig. 17-7. Unilateral **lymphoma of the palate.** (Courtesy Dr D. B. Smith)

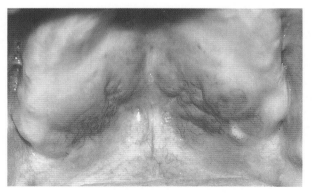

Fig. 17-8. Primary lymphoma of the palate appearing as a bilateral purplish swelling.

SWELLINGS OF THE FLOOR OF THE MOUTH

Dermoid Cyst (Figs. 18-1 and 18-2) The dermoid cyst is a soft tissue swelling derived from the cystic degeneration of epithelium entrapped during embryonic development. The cyst may occur anywhere on the skin, but has a propensity for the floor of the mouth. Although a small percentage appear very early in life, these cysts are more frequently seen in young adults under the age of 35. There is no sex predilection.

The dermoid cyst classically appears as a painless midline, dome-shaped mass arising in the floor of the mouth. The overlying mucosa is a natural pink, the tongue is slightly elevated, and palpation yields a dough-like consistency. Patients may complain of difficulties in eating and speaking. Growth of the cyst is slow, but diameters in excess of 5 cm may be seen. Dermoid cysts may appear below the floor of mouth if the original site of development is inferior to the mylohyoid muscle. In this instance a submental swelling is noted. Histologically the lesion is distinguished from an epidermoid cyst by the presence of adnexal structures in the fibrous wall such as sebaceous glands, sweat glands, and hair follicles. Dermoid cysts typically are lined with stratified squamous epithelium, but respiratory epithelium may also be present. The lumen contains semisolid keratin and sebum, which accounts for the doughy consistency and makes aspiration difficult. Surgical enucleation is the preferred treatment.

Ranula (Mucocele of the Sublingual Gland) (Figs. 18-3 and 18-4) The ranula is a large mucin-containing cyst in the floor of the mouth. It is identical to the mucous retention phenomenon except that the ranula is of greater size. The ranula forms as a result of inhibition of normal salivary flow through a dilated or severed major excretory duct of the sublingual gland (Bartholin's duct) or submandibular gland (Wharton's duct). No sex predilection is apparent, and persons under the age of 40 are most commonly affected.

There are two types of ranulae — the more common superficial ranula that appears as a soft compressible swelling rising up from the floor of the mouth, and the dissecting or plunging ranula that penetrates below the mylohyoid muscle to produce a submental swelling. The superficial ranula characteristically is translucent or has a bluish cast. It is unilateral, dome-shaped, and fluctuant. As the asymptomatic lesion enlarges, the mucosa becomes stretched, thinned, and tense. Digital pressure will not cause the lesion to pit, but rupture will cause the escape of mucous fluid. The entire floor of the mouth may be filled by the swelling, which elevates the tongue and hinders movement. This impairs mastication, deglutition, and speech.

A ranula can be differentiated from other floor-of-the-mouth swellings such as a dermoid cyst and mucoepidermoid carcinoma of the submandibular gland by sialography. Treatment is excision or marsupialization (Partsch operation), which consists of excising the regional mucosa and suturing the remaining cystic lining to the floor of the mouth. Incision and drainage is not the treatment of choice, since it will lead to reaccumulation of fluid as healing occurs. Recurrences are common in cases involving a plunging ranula or superficial ranula that is ill-managed. Removal of the affected major salivary gland is the indicated treatment for recurrent and plunging ranulae.

Salivary Calculi (Figs. 18-5 and 18-6) Sialoliths, also known a salivary calculi or stones, are concretions of calcium complexes within a salivary gland or duct that may obstruct salivary flow and cause floor-of-the-mouth swellings. Formation of stones occurs most frequently after the age of 25, twice as often in males as in females, and usually in the submandibular gland. The ascending course of the excretory duct, along with high mucous content and alkaline pH of the saliva, are significant factors in stone formation. Calculi are usually oval and smooth or irregularly surfaced.

Obstruction of salivary flow by a calculus results in a floor-of-the-mouth swelling that is firm, tender, and painful. Acute symptoms often recur at meal time. Swelling may extend along the course of the excretory duct and last for hours or days, depending on the blockage. The overlying mucosa usually remains pink. Secondary infection results in pus emanating from the ductal opening or in redness of the swollen floor of the mouth. Treatment involves appropriate occlusal radiographs, sialography (if no infection is present), and surgical removal of the sialolith. Localized cellulitis and fever require the use of antibiotics prior to invasive procedures.

Mucous Retention Phenomenon (Figs. 18-7 and 18-8) The mucous retention phenomenon is a soft fluctuant lesion involving the retention of mucous fluid in subepithelial tissue, usually as a result of trauma. These clear or bluish swellings may occur on the lip, floor of the mouth, ventral tongue, or buccal mucosa. They are usually asymptomatic and less than 1 cm in diameter. The base of the mucous retention phenomenon is commonly sessile, although pedunculated bases are possible. Children and young adults are most frequently affected. Treatment is excisional biopsy along with histopathologic examination. If the condition is managed properly, recurrences are rare.

SWELLINGS OF THE FLOOR OF THE MOUTH

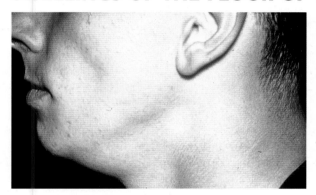

Fig. 18-1. Dermoid cyst protruding below the mylohyoid muscle.

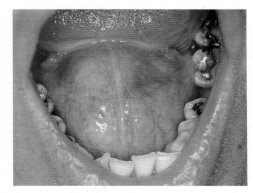

Fig. 18-2. Dermoid cyst appearing as a soft tissue swelling in the floor of the mouth.

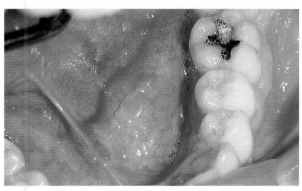

Fig. 18-3. Translucent fluctuant **ranula;** floor of the mouth.

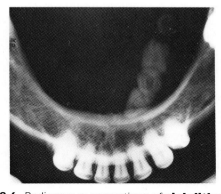

Fig. 18-4. Large **ranula** elevating the tongue. (Courtesy Dr Charles Morris)

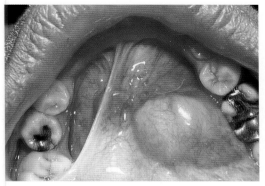

Fig. 18-5. Sialolith producing a firm and tender **floor-of-the-mouth swelling.**

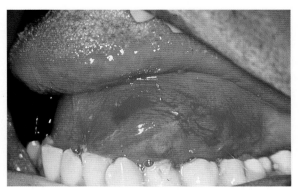

Fig. 18-6. Radiopaque concretions of **sialoliths** which obstructed salivary flow.

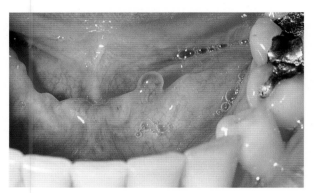

Fig. 18-7. Small polypoid **mucocele** on sublingual caruncle.

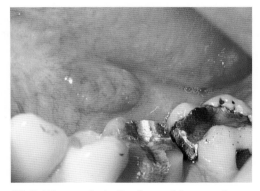

Fig. 18-8. Mucocele in the floor of the mouth caused by trauma during crown preparation.

CONDITIONS PECULIAR TO THE TONGUE

Normal Tongue Anatomy (Figs. 19-1 through 19-4) The tongue is a compact muscular organ covered by a protective layer of stratified squamous epithelium. It functions primarily in deglutition, taste, and speech. The dorsum of the tongue has numerous mucosal projections forming papillae. There are four types: filiform, fungiform, circumvallate, and foliate papillae. Filiform papillae are the smallest, but are also the most numerous. They are slender, hairlike, cornified stalks that may appear red, pink, or white, depending on the degree of daily irritation experienced. In contrast to filiform papillae, the fungiform papillae are fewer in number, brighter red in color, and broader in diameter; they also contain taste buds. Fungiform papillae are noncornified, round or mushroom-shaped, and slightly elevated. They are most numerous on the lateral border and anterior tip of the tongue. Occasionally fungiform papillae contain brown pigmentation, especially in melanoderms.

The largest papillae are the circumvallate papillae, which appear as 2- to 4-mm pink papules. They are surrounded by a narrow trench and also contain taste buds. These papillae are 8 to 12 in number and are arranged in a V-shaped row along the sulcus terminalis at the posterior aspect of the dorsum of the tongue. They anatomically divide the tongue into two unequal sections, the anterior two thirds and the posterior third.

If one looks carefully at the lateral border of the posterior region of the tongue the foliate papilla can be identified. These papillae are leaflike projections oriented as vertical folds. Occasionally, corrugated hypertrophic lymphoid tissue (lingual tonsil) extending into this area from the posterior dorsal root of the tongue may be mistakenly called foliate papillae. The plica fimbriata are linear projections on the ventral surface of the tongue. Sometimes the plica fimbriata have a brown pigmentation.

Fissured Tongue (Plicated Tongue, Scrotal Tongue) (Figs. 19-5 and 19-6) Fissured tongue is a variation of normal tongue anatomy that consists of a single midline fissure, double fissures, or multiple fissures of the dorsal surface of the anterior two thirds of the tongue. Various fissural patterns, lengths, and depths have been observed. The cause is unknown, but fissured tongue is probably developmental and increases with age.

Fissured tongue affects about 1 to 5% of the population.

The frequency of occurrence is equal between both sexes. Fissured tongue occurs commonly with Down's syndrome and in combination with geographic tongue. It is a component of the Melkerson-Rosenthal syndrome (fissured tongue, cheilitis granulomatosa, and unilateral facial nerve paralysis). The fissures may become secondarily inflamed and cause halitosis as a result of food impaction; therefore brushing the tongue to keep the fissures clean is recommended. The condition is benign.

Ankyloglossia (Fig. 19-7) The lingual frenum is normally attached to the ventral tongue and genial tubercles of the mandible. If the frenum fails to attach properly to the tongue and genial tubercles, but instead fuses to the floor of the mouth or lingual gingiva and the ventral tip of the tongue, the condition is called ankyloglossia, or "tongue-tie." This congenital condition is characterized by both an abnormally short and malpositioned lingual frenum and a tongue that cannot be extended or retracted. The fusion may be partial or complete. Partial fusion is more common. If the condition is severe, speech may be disturbed. Surgical correction and speech therapy are necessary if speech is defective, or if a mandibular denture or removable partial denture is planned. Ankyloglossia occurs with an estimated frequency of one case per 1000 births.

Lingual Varicosity (Phlebectasia) (Fig. 19-8) Lingual varicosities, or venous dilations, are a common finding in elderly adults. The etiology of these vascular dilitations is either a blockage of the vein by an internal foreign body, such as a plaque, or the loss of elasticity of the vascular wall as a result of aging. Intraoral varicosities most commonly appear superficially on the ventral surface of the anterior two thirds of the tongue and may extend onto the lateral border. Males and females are affected equally.

Varicosities appear as red-blue to purple, fluctuant nodular growths. Individual varices may be prominent and tortuous, or small and punctate. Palpation elicits no pain, but can disperse the blood from the vessel, flattening the surface appearance. When many lingual veins are prominent the condition is called "phlebectasia linguae" or "caviar tongue." The lip and labial commissure are other frequent sites of phlebectasia. No treatment is required of this condition.

CONDITIONS PECULIAR TO THE TONGUE

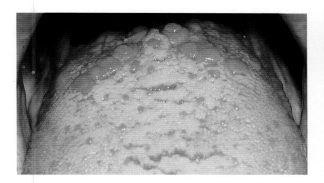

Fig. 19-1. Large pink **circumvallate papillae** forming a 'V'-shaped row. (Courtesy Dr James Cottone)

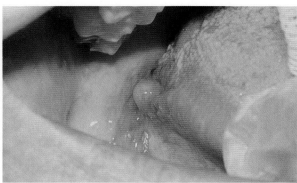

Fig. 19-2. Foliate papilla on the lateral border of the tongue.

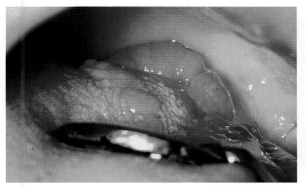

Fig. 19-3. Lingual tonsil apparent posterior to the circumvallate papillae.

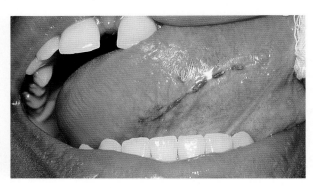

Fig. 19-4. Plica fimbriata which is pigmented in this individual.

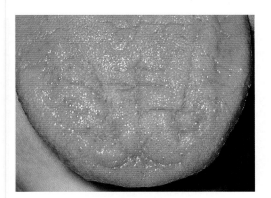

Fig. 19-5. Fissured tongue, a mild case.

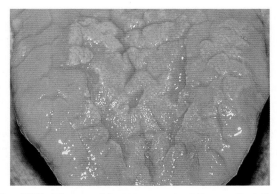

Fig. 19-6. Fissured tongue and subtle manifestations of geographic tongue.

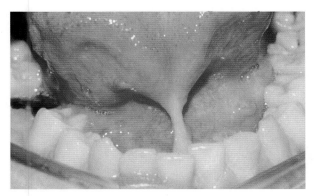

Fig. 19-7. Ankyloglossia.

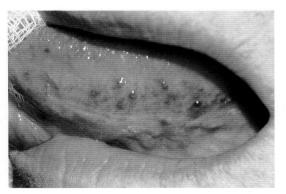

Fig. 19-8. Multiple purple lingual **varicosities;** ventral tongue. (Courtesy Dr Linda Otis)

43

CONDITIONS PECULIAR TO THE TONGUE

Scalloped Tongue (Crenated Tongue) (Figs. 20-1 and 20-2) A scalloped tongue is a common entity characterized by indentations on the lateral margins of the tongue. The condition is usually bilateral, but may be unilateral or isolated to a region where the tongue is held in close contact with the teeth. Abnormal pressure of the teeth on the tongue imprints the characteristic pattern, which appears as depressed ovals that are circumscribed by a raised white scalloped border. Causes of scalloped tongue include situations that cause abnormal tongue pressure such as frictional movement of the tongue against teeth and diastemata, tongue thrusting, tongue sucking, clenching, or an enlarged tongue. A crenated tongue may be seen in association with temporomandibular joint disorders, systemic conditions such as acromegaly and amyloidosis, and genetic disorders such as Down's syndrome, as well as in normal patients. The condition is harmless and asymptomatic. Treatment is often aimed at habit elimination.

Macroglossia (Figs. 20-3 and 20-4) Macroglossia is the term used to indicate an abnormally enlarged tongue. To assess tongue size, the tongue should be completely relaxed. The normal height of the dorsum of the tongue should be even with the occlusal plane of the mandibular teeth; the lateral borders of the tongue should be in contact with, but not overlapping, the lingual cusps of the mandibular teeth. A tongue that extends beyond these dimensions is said to be enlarged.

Macroglossia is either congenital or acquired. Congenital macroglossia can be caused by idiopathic muscular hypertrophy, muscular hemihypertrophy, benign tumors, hamartomas, or cysts. Idiopathic muscular hypertrophy is often associated with a mental deficiency, or may be a component of a syndrome such as Beckwith-Wiedemann's syndrome. Acquired macroglossia may be the result of passive enlargement of the tongue when mandibular teeth are lost. In this case the enlargement may be localized or diffuse, depending on the size of the edentulous area. Systemic disease such as acromegaly, cretinism, and amyloidosis, or malignant neoplasms, which can occlude lymphatic drainage and produce a swollen tongue, can cause macroglossia. Indicators of an enlarged tongue are speech difficulties, displaced teeth, malocclusion, or a scalloped tongue. Often the affected region of the tongue demonstrates enlarged fungiform papillae. If the enlarged tongue is hindering function, elimination of the primary cause and/or surgical correction is recommended.

Hairy Tongue (Lingua Villosa, Coated Tongue) (Figs. 20-5 and 20-6) Hairy tongue is an abnormal elongation of the filiform papillae that gives the dorsum of the tongue a hairlike appearance. The cause of the hypertrophic response of the filiform papillae is poorly understood but seems to be related to either increased keratin deposition or delayed shedding of the cornified layer. Patients who fail to cleanse their tongues are most commonly affected. Cancer therapy, infection with *Candida albicans,* irradiation, poor oral hygiene, change in oral pH, smoking, and the use of antibiotics have also been associated with this condition.

Hairy tongue may be white, yellow, brown, or black; hence the names white coated tongue and yellow, brown, or black hairy tongue. The color of the lesion is a result of intrinsic factors (chromogenic organisms) combined with extrinsic factors (food and tobacco stains). Hairy tongue occurs more frequently in males, primarily in persons over the age of 30, and the prevalence seems to increase with age. The lesion begins near the foramen cecum on the dorsal surface of the tongue and spreads laterally and anteriorly. The affected filiform papillae discolor, progressively elongate, and may reach a length of several millimeters. Usually the tongue remains asymptomatic, but severe cases may become uncomfortable because of pruritis. Generally, hairy tongue is only of cosmetic concern. Vigorous brushing with abrasive pastes and topical antifungal agents leads to resolution. In cases that are refractory an underlying endocrinopathy such as diabetes mellitus should be sought.

Hairy Leukoplakia (Figs. 20-7 and 20-8) Hairy leukoplakia is a significant leukoplakic-like finding that indicates human immune deficiency virus (HIV; HTLV-III) infection and immunosuppression. This lesion is primarily located on the lateral borders of the tongue, but may extend to cover the dorsal and ventral surfaces. A viral origin is likely since Epstein-Barr virus has been identified within the affected epithelial cells. Hairy leukoplakia is so named because hair-like peeling of the parakeratotic surface layer is evident histologically. *Candida albicans* is frequently associated with this lesion.

Hairy leukoplakia produces white vertical raised folds on the lateral border of the tongue. Initially the lesion has alternating faint white folds and adjacent normal pink troughs that produce a characteristic vertical white-banded washboard appearance. The bands eventually coalesce to form discrete white plaques or extensive thick white corrugated patches. Large lesions are usually asymptomatic, have poorly demarcated borders, and do not rub off. A bilateral occurrence is common, but unilateral lesions are a possibility. Hairy leukoplakic lesions have been documented on the palate and buccal mucosa. Antiviral agents may reduce the size of the lesion, but do little to alter the course of HIV infection.

CONDITIONS PECULIAR TO THE TONGUE

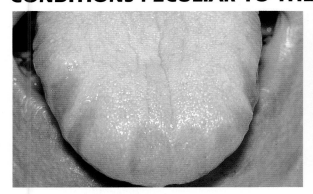

Fig. 20-1. Scalloped tongue caused by abnormal tongue pressure against the teeth.

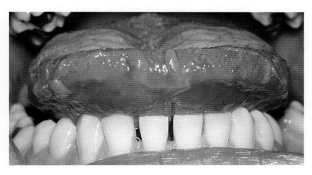

Fig. 20-2. Localized **scalloping** due to tongue sucking.

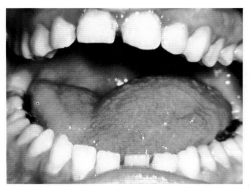

Fig. 20-3. Hemihypertrophic tongue.

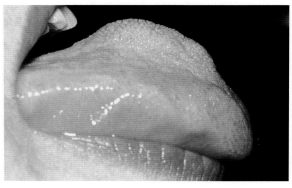

Fig. 20-4. Macroglossia due to a hemangioma. (Courtesy Dr Kenneth Abramovitch)

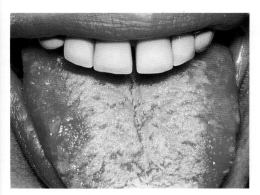

Fig. 20-5. White hairy tongue.

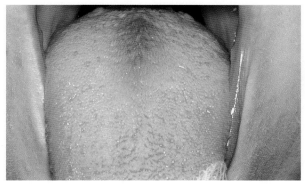

Fig. 20-6. Brown hairy tongue in an individual that smokes.

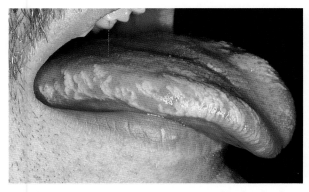

Fig. 20-7. Extensive white corrugations of **hairy leukoplakia** in a patient with AIDS. (Courtesy Dr Sol Silverman)

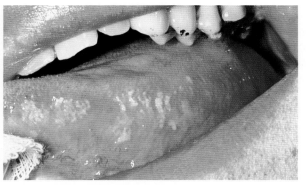

Fig. 20-8. Hairy leukoplakia in an individual who just received dental treatment. (Courtesy Dr Micheal Huber)

CONDITIONS PECULIAR TO THE TONGUE

Geographic Tongue (Benign Migratory Glossitis, Erythema Migrans, Wandering Rash) (Figs. 21-1 through 21-6) Geographic tongue is a benign inflammatory condition caused by desquamation of superficial keratin and the filiform papillae. The etiology is unknown, but emotional stress, nutritional deficiencies, and heredity have been suggested. The condition is usually restricted to the dorsal and lateral borders of the anterior two thirds of the tongue, affecting only the filiform papillae and leaving the fungiform papillae intact.

Geographic tongue is characterized by single or multiple pink to red denuded patches of desquamated filiform papillae that may or may not be bordered by a raised white serpiginous rim. An adjacent red band of inflammation at the leading edge of the lesion may be concurrent. When inflammation is present, pain is often a feature. The lesion continuously changes patterns and migrates from site to site; hence the synonymous name "benign migratory glossitis," "erythema migrans," and "wandering rash."

Geographic tongue is common, affecting approximately 1 to 2% of the population. Females and young to middle-aged adults are most frequently affected. The condition may appear suddenly and persist for months or years. Spontaneous remissions and recurrences have been observed. Geographic tongue is occasionally seen in association with a mucosal counterpart, areata erythema migrans (migratory mucositis, geographic stomatitis, ectopic geographic tongue), and fissured tongue. Erythema migrans, when asymptomatic, is harmless and requires no treatment. More often than not, erythema migrans produces red annular patches that burn. Topical anesthetics or topical steroids may be given to the symptomatic patient. Histologically this lesion resembles psoriasis; however, it is generally accepted that these conditions are distinct entities, though they may sometimes co-exist.

Anemia (Fig. 21-7) Anemia is a condition of impaired oxygen delivery to bodily tissues that results from a deficiency in red blood cells, hemoglobin, or total blood volume. Underlying causes of anemia include increased destruction of red blood cells due to hemolysis, increased blood loss due to hemorrhage, or a decreased production of red blood cells due to a nutritional deficiency state or bone marrow suppression. Anemia is not a final diagnosis, but a sign of an underlying disease; thus the cause of anemia must always be sought. Iron deficiency is the most common type of anemia, frequently affecting middle-aged women and young teenagers. Deficiencies in vitamin B_{12} and folic acid will also cause anemia and produce oral signs of the condition.

Anemia produces characteristic changes in the appearance of the oral mucous membranes. These manifestations, although suggestive of anemia, are not helpful in distiguishing the type of anemia causing the features seen. Analysis of red blood cell morphology is recommended for a more accurate diagnosis.

Intraoral manifestations of anemia are most prominent on the tongue. The dorsum of the tongue initially appears pale, with flattening of the filiform papillae. Continued atrophy of the papillae results in a surface devoid of papillae that appears smooth, dry, and glazed. This condition is commonly referred to as "bald tongue." In the final stage, a beefy or fiery red tongue is seen, possibly with concurrent oral aphthae.

Anemic patients may complain of a sore, painful tongue (glossodynia) or burning tongue (glossopyrosis). The lips may be thinned and taut, while the width of the mouth may develop a narrowed appearance. Other clinical signs associated with anemia include angular cheilitis, aphthous ulceration, dysphagia, mucosal erythema and erosions, pallor, shortness of breath, fatigue, dizziness, and a bounding pulse. Patients with a vitamin B_{12} deficiency may complain of weight loss, weakness, neurological disturbances such as numbness and tingling of the extremities, and difficulty in walking. Therapy should be directed toward correcting the underlying cause. Improvement after therapy is reflected in changes in the oral appearance.

Xerostomia (Fig. 21-8) Saliva functions to keep the oral cavity moist and aids in mastication, deglutition, digestion, speech, and immunologic neutralization. When impaired salivary function causes a dry mouth the condition is called xerostomia. Manifestations of decreased salivary flow can be subtle with no patient complaints, or severe with a myriad of complaints. Xerostomia may result from advancing age, anemia, avitaminosis, dehydration, diabetes, emotional stress, mechanical blockage, surgery, collagen vascular disease, ectodermal dysplasia, mumps, Mikulicz's disease, multiple sclerosis, Sjogren's syndrome, acquired immunodeficiency syndrome, and head and neck irradiation. Many therapeutic drugs, principally antidepressants, antihistamines, antihypertensive and cardiac agents, decongestants, ganglionic blocking agents, and tranquilizers will also produce xerostomia.

Mild cases of xerostomia are relatively free of symptoms, and the mucosa appears normal. In moderate cases the tongue is dry, pale, red, and atrophic, with its dorsal surface wrinkled or smooth. In severe situations the tongue may be devoid of papillae, fissured, and inflamed. The mucosa appears dry, shiny, and sticky, while the lips appear cracked and fissured. Stagnant, rope-like accumulations of saliva on the tongue along with burning tongue (glossopyrosis) and alterations in taste are usually present. Progression of xerostomia can result in halitosis, multiple carious lesions evident at the gingival tooth margin, and difficulty with speech, mastication, and retention of prosthodontic appliances. Chronic xerostomia requires long term multiphasic support, including such items as emollients, artificial saliva, pilocarpine, fluoride treatment, oral hygiene instructions, and nutritional counseling.

CONDITIONS PECULIAR TO THE TONGUE

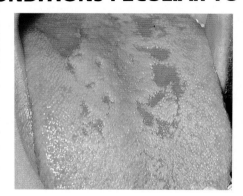

Fig. 21-1. Pink-red denudations of filiform papillae typical of mild **geographic tongue.**

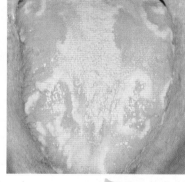

Fig. 21-2. Extensive case of **geographic tongue** with white circinate borders. (Courtesy Dr Bill Baker)

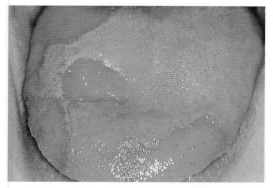

Fig. 21-3. Symptomatic **geographic tongue** exhibiting mild inflammatory borders.

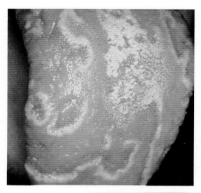

Fig. 21-4. Symptomatic **geographic tongue** with a prominent red-white inflammatory border.

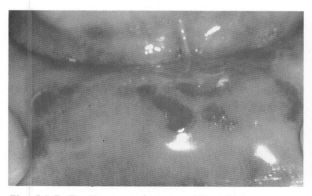

Fig. 21-5. Erythema migrans of the labial mucosa.

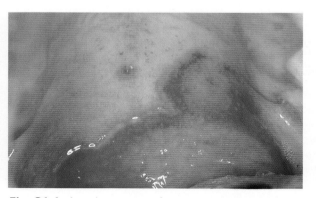

Fig. 21-6. Annular pattern of symptomatic **erythema migrans** of the hard and soft palate.

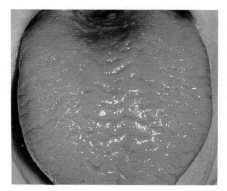

Fig. 21-7. Smooth, bald, burning tongue; **iron deficiency anemia.**

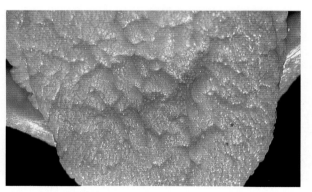

Fig. 21-8. Xerostomia-induced dry, fissured atrophic tongue. (Courtesy Dr Pete Benson)

CONDITIONS PECULIAR TO THE TONGUE

Median Rhomboid Glossitis (Central Papillary Atrophy of the Tongue) (Figs. 22-1 through 22-4) Median rhomboid glossitis was once thought to be a developmental defect of incomplete descent of the tuberculum impar. Recently this theory has fallen into disfavor; it is now believed that median rhomboid glossitis is a permanent end result of a *Candida albicans* infection in conjunction with other factors (possibly smoking or a change in oral pH). Median rhomboid glossitis frequently affects middle-aged adult males and rarely affects children. Blacks and whites are affected equally. Diabetics, immune-suppressed patients, and patients who recently completed a course of broad spectrum antibiotics have a higher prevalence of this condition.

Median rhomboid glossitis is a smooth, denuded, beefy red patch devoid of filiform papillae. With time the lesion becomes granular, lobular, and indurated. The most common location is the midline of the dorsum of the tongue, just anterior to the circumvallate papillae. The size and shape of the lesion varies, but it frequently appears as a well-demarcated 1 to 2.5 cm oval or rhomboid with irregular but rounded borders. The condition is generally asymptomatic. Occasionally an erythematous palatal candidal lesion is observed directly over the lesion of the tongue.

Median rhomboid glossitis is easily recognized by its clinical appearance, characteristic location, and asymptomatic nature. Early recognition and treatment with antimonilial agents may lead to resolution. End-stage median rhomboid glossitis is usually asymptomatic but refractory to antifungal treatment. The rare possibility of anaplastic transformation exists.

Granular Cell Tumor (Granular Cell Myoblastoma) (Figs. 22-5 and 22-6) The granular cell tumor is a rare benign soft-tissue tumor composed of oval cells that have an extremely granular cytoplasm. This tumor may occur in a variety of cutaneous, mucosal, and visceral sites, but its favorite oral site of occurrence is the dorsal-lateral surface of the tongue. Theories of histogenesis have been controversial. Most investigators believe that the tumor is actually a benign proliferation of neurogenic cells.

The granular cell tumor can occur at any age and in any race, but it has a slight predilection for females. Usually the lesion consists of a symptomless, solitary, dome-shaped submucosal nodule covered clinically by normal, yellow, or white tissue. The surface may be ulcerated when it has been traumatized. The granular cell tumor is often sessile, well-circumscribed, and firm to compression. Growth is very slow and painless, with some tumors achieving several centimeters in size. Larger lesions may demonstrate a slightly depressed central area. Rarely these lesions are found on the ventral surface of the tongue. Approximately 10% of affected patients experience multiple lesions.

The granular cell tumor is characterized by pseudoepitheliomatous hyperplasia and granular cells that may histologically resemble epidermoid carcinoma and the congenital epulis of the newborn, respectively. Conservative local excision is the preferred treatment, and these lesions do not tend to recur.

Lingual Thyroid (Fig. 22-7) Lingual thyroid is an uncommon nodule of thyroid tissue found just posterior to the foramen cecum on the posterior third of the tongue. It occurs when embryonic tissue from the thyroid gland fails to migrate to the anterolateral surface of the trachea. Persistent thyroid tissue occurs much more frequently in women than in men (the ratio is 4:1) and may appear at any age. If the remnant tissue becomes cystic the condition becomes a thyroglossal duct cyst.

The lingual thyroid is a raised asymptomatic mass that usually measures about 2 cm in diameter. Increased surface vascularity is a prominent feature. Hemorrhage, dysphagia, dysphonia, symptoms of hypothyroidism, and (rarely) pain can be associated with the condition. The lesion may be differentiated from similar lesions by confirming its distinctive location posterior to the circumvallate papillae and by utilizing radionuclide studies. Biopsy should be deferred until it is ascertained that the remainder of the thyroid gland is present and functioning. In over 50% of patients with ectopic thyroid the lingual thyroid is the only active thyroid tissue present.

Cyst of Blandin-Nuhn (Lingual Mucous Retention Cyst) (Fig. 22-8) The glands of Blandin-Nuhn are the accessory salivary glands on the ventral surface of the tongue composed of mixed serous and mucous elements. When trauma of the ventral tongue induces extravasation of saliva into the surrounding tissues, a relatively small painless swelling develops, which is termed the cyst of Blandin-Nuhn. This infrequent accessory salivary gland cyst is located near the tip of the ventral surface of the tongue. The borders are raised and well-demarcated, the mucosal surface appears pink-red, and the lesion is soft and fluctuant. When superficial, the cyst has balloon-like features and a pedunculated base. Deeper lesions have sessile bases. Although usually traumatically induced, the cyst of Blandin-Nuhn may be congenital. These cysts rarely exceed 1 cm in diameter. Treatment is excisional biopsy, and recurrence is rare.

CONDITIONS PECULIAR TO THE TONGUE

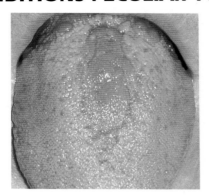

Fig. 22-1. Hypertrophic **median rhomboid glossitis.**

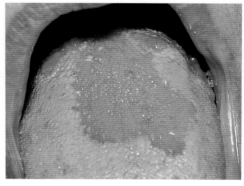

Fig. 22-2. Smooth denuded patch with irregular borders; **median rhomboid glossitis.** (Courtesy Dr Linda Otis)

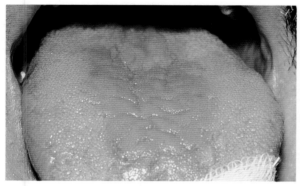

Fig. 22-3. Central area of tongue devoid of filiform papillae characteristic of **median rhomboid glossitis.**

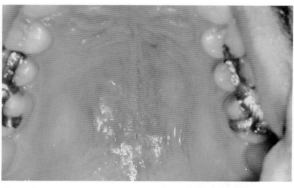

Fig. 22-4. Red palatal lesion of **atrophic candidiasis** directly overlying median rhomboid glossitis seen in Fig. 22-3.

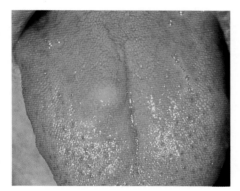

Fig. 22-5. Granular cell tumor appearing as a pink tongue nodule. (Courtesy Dr Jerry Cioffi)

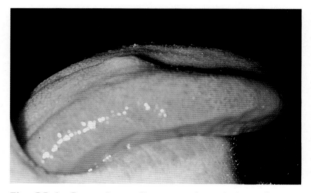

Fig. 22-6. Granular cell tumor; lateral view of same patient as in Fig. 22-5. (Courtesy Dr Jerry Cioffi)

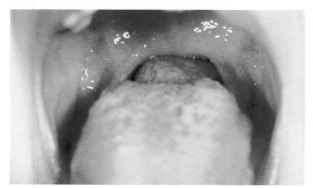

Fig. 22-7. Vascular **lingual thyroid;** posterior to the sulcus terminalis. (Courtesy Dr Tom Aufdemorte)

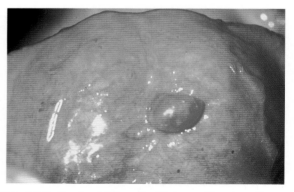

Fig. 22-8. Cyst of Blandin-Nuhn. (Courtesy Dr James Cottone)

IV

Intraoral Findings by Color Changes

WHITE LESIONS

Fordyce's Granules (Figs. 23-1 and 23-2) Fordyce's granules are ectopic sebaceous glands found within the mouth that are considered a variation of normal oral mucosal anatomy. These granules consist of individual sebaceous glands that are 1 to 2 mm in diameter. Characteristically they appear on the buccal mucosa as white, creamy white, or yellow slightly raised papules. They usually occur in multiples, forming clusters, plaques, or patches. Clusters that are enlarged may feel rough to palpation. Occasionally they are an isolated finding. Less common locations include the lip, labial mucosa, retromolar pad, attached gingiva, tongue, and frenum.

Fordyce's granules arise from sebaceous glands embryologically entrapped during fusion of the maxillary and mandibular processes. They become more apparent after sexual maturity as the sebaceous system develops. Rarely an intraoral hair may be seen in association with the condition.

Fordyce's granules occur in approximately 80% of adults, and no predilection in race or sex has been reported. Histologically, rounded nests of clear cells, 10 to 30 per nest, with darkly staining, small, centrally located nuclei are found encapsulated in the lamina propria and submucosa. The clinical appearance is adequate for diagnosis of Fordyce's granules; biopsy is not usually required.

Linea Alba Buccalis (Figs. 23-3 and 23-4) The linea alba buccalis is a common intraoral finding that appears as a raised white wavy line of variable length located at the level of the occlusion on the buccal mucosa. Generally this asymptomatic cornified entity is 1 to 2 mm in width and extends from the second molar to the canine region of the buccal mucosa. The lesion is usually found bilaterally and cannot be rubbed off. The thickened epithelial changes consist of hyperkeratotic tissue that is a response to frictional activity of the teeth. The condition is often associated with crenated tongue and may be a sign of bruxism, clenching, or negative oral pressure. The clinical appearance is diagnostic and requires no treatment.

Leukoedema (Figs. 23-5 and 23-6) Leukoedema is a common mucosal variant associated with dark-pigmented individuals, but may be seen infrequently in lighter-pigmented persons. The incidence of leukoedema tends to increase with age, and 50% of black children and 92% of adult blacks are affected. Leukoedema usually appears bilaterally on the buccal mucosa as an opalescent, white, or gray thin surface film. The labial mucosa and soft palate are less common locations of occurrence.

Leukoedema is often faint and may be difficult to see. Prominence of the lesion is related to the degree of underlying melanin pigmentation, level of oral hygiene, and amount of smoking. Close examination of leukoedema reveals fine white lines, wrinkles, or overlapping folds of tissue. The borders of the lesion are irregular and diffuse; they fade into adjacent tissue making it difficult to determine where the lesion begins and ends. Diagnosis is obtained by stretching the mucosa, causing the white appearance to significantly diminish or disappear in some cases. Wiping the lesion fails to remove it. The etiology of leukoedema is unknown. No serious complications are associated with this lesion, nor is treatment required.

Morsicatio Buccarum (Mucosal Chewing) (Figs. 23-7 and 23-8) Morsicatio buccarum, or cheek biting, is a common habit that produces a progression of mucosal changes. Initially, slightly raised white plaques and folds appear in a diffuse pattern covering areas of trauma. Increased injury produces a hyperplastic response that increases the size of the plaque. A linear or striated pattern is sometimes observed, with thick and thin areas seen side-by-side. Persistent injury leads to interadjacent traumatic erythema and ulceration.

Mucosal chewing is usually seen on the buccal mucosa, less frequently on the labial mucosa. The lesions may be unilateral or bilateral and can occur at any age. No sex or race predilection has been reported. Diagnosis requires visual or verbal confirmation of the nervous habit. Although morsicatio buccarum has no malignant potential, patients should be advised of the mucosal alterations. Because of the similar clinical appearance, speckled leukoplakia and candidiasis should be ruled out. Microscopically there is a normal maturing epithelial surface with a corrugated parakeratotic surface and minor subepithelial inflammation.

WHITE LESIONS

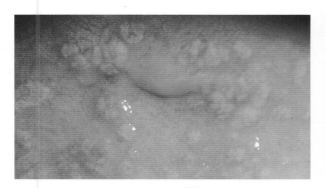

Fig. 23-1. Multiple creamy white **fordyce granules** on buccal mucosa. (Courtesy Dr Linda Otis)

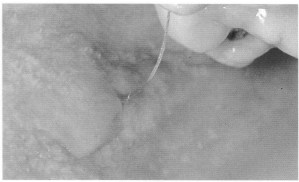

Fig. 23-2. Clusters of **fordyce granules** with a rare intraoral hair. (Courtesy Dr Bill Baker)

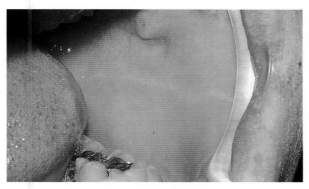

Fig. 23-3. White wavy **linea alba buccalis.**

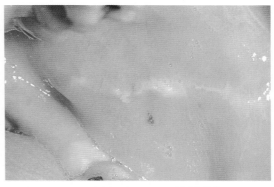

Fig. 23-4. Keratotic **linea alba buccalis** with mild leukoedema. (Courtesy Dr Dale Miles)

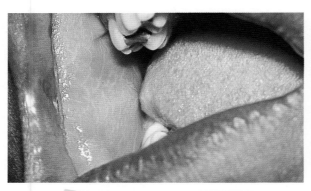

Fig. 23-5. Leukoedema of the buccal mucosa in a melanoderm.

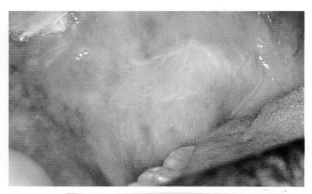

Fig. 23-6. Patch-like distribution of **leukoedema;** buccal mucosa.

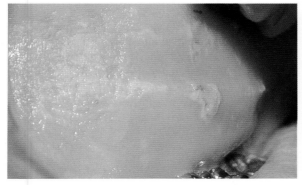

Fig. 23-7. Cheek biting producing white plaques characteristic of **morsicatio buccarum.**

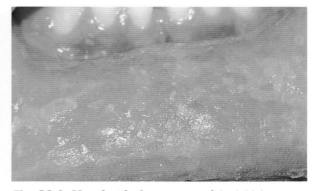

Fig. 23-8. Morsicatio buccarum of the labial mucosa. (Courtesy Dr Kenneth Abramovitch)

WHITE LESIONS

White Sponge Nevus (Familial White Folded Dysplasia) (Figs. 24-1 and 24-2)
White sponge nevus is a relatively uncommon entity that usually appears at birth or in early childhood but persists throughout life. It is characterized by mucosal lesions that are asymptomatic, white, folded, and spongy. Often the lesions exhibit a symmetric wavy pattern. The most common location is the buccal mucosa, bilaterally, followed by the labial mucosa, alveolar ridge, and floor of the mouth. This condition may involve the entire oral mucosa, or may be distributed unilaterally as discrete white patches. The gingival margin and dorsal tongue are almost never affected, although the soft palate and ventral tongue are commonly involved. The size of the lesions varies from patient to patient and from time to time.

White sponge nevus exhibits no race, sex or gender predilection; however, because of this condition's autosomal dominant pattern of transmission, multiple family members may manifest the disorder. Extraoral mucosal sites may involve the nasal cavity, esophagus, larynx, vagina, and rectum. Concurrent skin lesions exclude the diagnosis. Causation has been attributed to a basic defect in epithelial maturation and exfoliation. No treatment is required, and the lesions are harmless.

Traumatic White Lesions (Acute Trauma, Chemical Burns and Peripheral Scar) (Figs. 24-3 through 24-6)
Traumatic white lesions can be caused by a variety of physical and chemical irritants such as frictional trauma, heat, prolonged aspirin contact, and excessive use of mouthwash or other caustic liquids. In particular, frictional trauma is often noted on the attached gingiva. It is caused by excessive tooth brushing, movement of oral prostheses, and chewing on the edentulous ridge. With time the mucosa becomes thickened with a roughened white surface. Pain is characteristically absent, and histologic examination reveals hyperorthokeratosis.

Severe trauma can produce a white lesion owing to the loss of the superficial layers of mucosal epithelium. Underneath the white slough there is a raw, red, or bleeding surface. Typically acute traumatic lesions appear as punctate white patches with diffuse and irregular borders. Moveable mucosa is more susceptible to trauma than attached mucosa. Pain of several days duration is common.

Trauma involving the subjacent dermal layers may induce a fibrous healing response or scar. Scars are often asymptomatic, linear, pale pink, and sharply delineated. A thorough history may reveal previous injury, recurrent ulcerative disease, seizure disorder, self-multilating behavior, or previous surgery.

Leukoplakia (Figs. 24-7 and 24-8)
Leukoplakia is a clinical term descriptive for a white plaque or patch on the oral mucosa that cannot be scraped off and cannot be classified as any other clinically diagnosable disease. Individuals of any age may be affected; however, the majority of cases occur in men between the ages of 45 and 65. Recent incidence figures indicate that the male to female ratio is decreasing, with women being affected almost as frequently as men.

Leukoplakias are protective reactions against chronic irritants. Tobacco, alcohol, syphilis, vitamin deficiency, hormonal imbalance, galvanism, chronic friction, and candidiasis have been implicated in the cause of these lesions. Leukoplakias vary considerably in size, location, and clinical appearance. The preferential sites for leukoplakia are the lateral and ventral tongue, floor of mouth, alveolar mucosa, lip, soft palate-retromolar trigone, and mandibular attached gingiva. The lesional surface may appear smooth and homogeneous, thin and friable, fissured, corrugated, verrucoid, nodular, or speckled. The color can take on subtle variations from faintly translucent white lesions to gray or brown-white.

A classification system offered by the World Health Organization (WHO) recommends two divisions for oral leukoplakias: homogeneous and nonhomogeneous. Nonhomogeneous leukoplakias have been further subdivided into erythroleukoplakia, nodular, speckled, and verrucoid.

The majority of leukoplakias (80%) are benign; the remaining cases are dysplastic or cancerous. The clinical dilemma is in determining which leukoplakias are premalignant or malignant, especially since 4 to 6% of all leukoplakias progress to squamous cell carcinoma within 5 years. High risk sites for malignancy include the floor of the mouth, lateral and ventral tongue, uvulo-palatal complex, and lips.

Leukoplakias with localized red areas also confer a high risk of carcinoma. For example, nonhomogeneous leukoplakias, particularly oral speckled leukoplakias, represent epithelial dysplasia in about half of the cases and have the highest rate of malignant transformation among intraoral leukoplakias. Candida albicans, a fungal organism often associated with oral speckled leukoplakias, may have a role in the dysplastic changes seen.

The initial step in the treatment of leukoplakia is to eliminate any irritating and causative factors, then observe for healing. The lesion may or may not disappear. When an unexplained oral leukoplakia is persistent, biopsy is mandatory. Multiple biopsy sites may be necessary for diffuse lesions. Nonhomogeneous areas of the lesion should always be selected for biopsy.

WHITE LESIONS

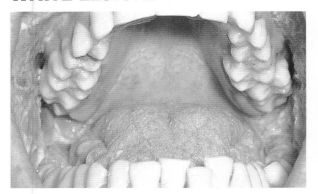

Fig. 24-1. White sponge nevus affecting the buccal mucosa, soft palate, and retromolar pad.

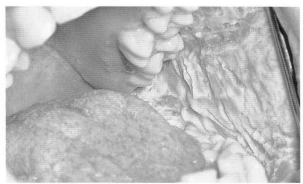

Fig. 24-2. Thick white plaques of **white sponge nevus** in same patient shown in Fig. 24-1. Gingival margin remains unaffected.

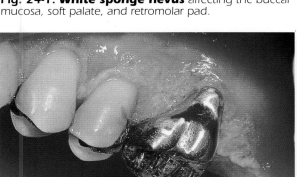

Fig. 24-3. Frictional keratosis associated with vigorous tooth brushing.

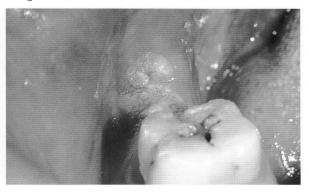

Fig. 24-4. White pebbly **frictional keratosis** from traumatic occlusion.

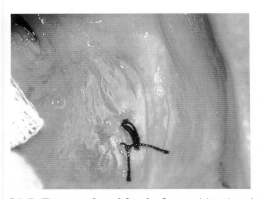

Fig. 24-5. Traumatic white lesion; white chemical burn from aspirin placement at a biopsy site.

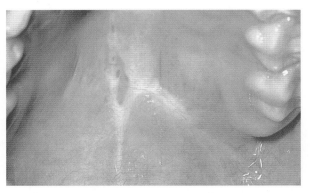

Fig. 24-6. Traumatic laceration at age 2 resulted in this palatal **scar.**

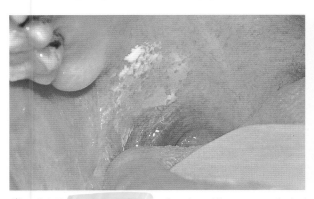

Fig. 24-7. Leukoplakia; soft palate. Biopsy revealed hyperorthokeratosis.

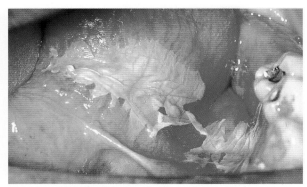

Fig. 24-8. Leukoplakia of the floor of the mouth and ventral tongue; biopsy revealed mild epithelial dysplasia.

TOBACCO ASSOCIATED WHITE LESIONS

Cigarette Keratosis (Figs. 25-1 and 25-2)
Cigarette keratosis is a specific reaction evident in individuals who smoke non-filtered or marijuana cigarettes to a very short length. The lesions, which approximate each other upon lip closure, involve both the upper and lower lip at the location of cigarette placement. These keratotic patches are about 7 mm in diameter and invariably are located lateral to the midline. Raised white papules are evident throughout the patch, producing a roughened texture and firmness to palpation. Occasionally cigarette keratoses may extend onto the labial mucosa, but rarely is the vermilion border involved. Elderly males are most commonly affected. Discontinuation of the smoking habit usually brings about resolution. The development of ulcer and crust formation should raise the suspicion of neoplastic transformation.

Nicotine Stomatitis (Pipe Smoker's Palate) (Figs. 25-3 and 25-4) Nicotine stomatitis is a response of palatal ectodermal structures to prolonged pipe and cigar smoking. Usually found in middle-aged and elderly males, posterior to the palatal rugae, this lesion shows progressive changes with time. Initially the irritation causes the palate to become diffusely erythematous. Eventually the palate becomes grayish-white secondary to hyperkeratosis. Multiple discrete keratotic papules with depressed red centers develop that correspond to dilated and inflamed minor salivary gland excretory duct openings. The papules enlarge as the irritation persists but fail to coalesce, producing a characteristic cobblestone (parboiled) appearance of the palate. Isolated but prominent red-centered papules are common. Whether the lesion arises as a consequence of heat or of tobacco is a matter of debate. Reverse cigarette smoking produces similar findings. Discontinuation of smoking should result in regression.

Snuff Dipper's Patch (Tobacco Chewer's Lesion, Snuff Keratosis) (Figs. 25-5 and 25-6) A wrinkled yellow-white area on the gingival mucosal flexure and mandibular buccal or labial mucosa is indicative of intraoral use of unburned tobacco. Smokeless tobacco may take various forms (snuff, dip, plug, or quid), leaving its characteristic mark at the preferential site of tobacco placement. Posterior sites are commonly utilized for dip, plug, or quid, whereas anterior sites are preferential for snuff. Individuals who vary intraoral sites have multiple, less prominent lesions. Male teenagers are most frequently affected, largely because of intensive marketing efforts by tobacco companies.

Early snuff dipper's patches are pale pink in color, with the surface appearing corrugated and wrinkled. A progression to white, yellow-white, and yellow-brown may ensue as hyperkeratosis and exogenous staining occur.

Chronic smokeless tobacco use is associated with periodontal alterations, caries, epidermal dysplastic changes, and verrucous carcinoma. To achieve resolution, cessation of use is recommended. If normal appearance does not return 14 days after cessation, biopsy is necessary.

Verrucous Carcinoma (of Ackerman) (Oral Florid Papillomatosis) (Figs. 25-7 and 25-8) This warty, exophytic, cauliflower-like whitish mass is a variant malignant squamous cell tumor that is considered low-grade and nonmetastasizing. The buccal mucosa and mandibular gingiva are the most common locations. Males over 60 years of age who use smokeless tobacco are most often affected. The disease is rare in persons under 40 years of age.

Verrucous carcinoma has a distinctive surface appearance. Characteristically there is a white keratotic surface with pink-red pebbly papules throughout. Lateral growth leads to an increase in mass, and the tumor can achieve several centimeters or more in diameter. Large lesions can be locally destructive by invading and eroding the underlying alveolar bone. Similar-appearing lesions include verrucous epithelial hyperplasia, pyostomatitis vegetans, and proliferating verrucous leukoplakia.

Recommended treatment is wide surgical excision. Radiation therapy is contraindicated, since there is a risk of anaplastic transformation to squamous cell carcinoma.

TOBACCO ASSOCIATED WHITE LESIONS

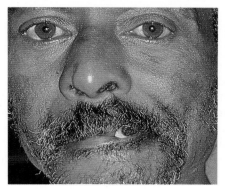

Fig. 25-1. 65-year-old male with cigarette smoking habit and **cigarette keratosis.**

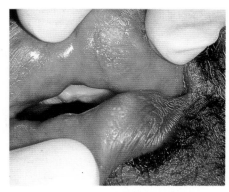

Fig. 25-2. Cigarette keratosis on labial mucosa of patient in Fig. 25-1.

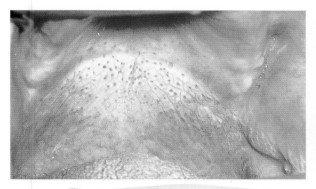

Fig. 25-3. Nicotine stomatitis prominent on the soft palate, extending onto the buccal mucosa.

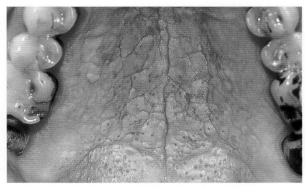

Fig. 25-4. Cobblestone appearance of **nicotine stomatitis** in a reverse smoker.

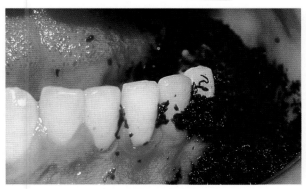

Fig. 25-5. Typical placement of chewing tobacco, which causes a **snuff dipper's patch.**

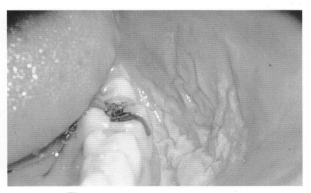

Fig. 25-6. Wrinkled appearance of a **snuff dipper's patch.**

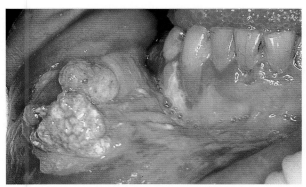

Fig. 25-7. Fungating **verrucous carcinoma** of the labial mucosa after many years of tobacco chewing. (Courtesy Dr Spencer Redding)

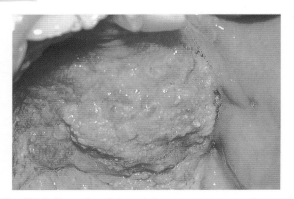

Fig. 25-8. Extensive pink nodular **verrucous carcinoma**; alveolar ridge and palate. (Courtesy Dr James Cottone)

RED LESIONS

Purpura (Petechiae, Ecchymoses, Hematoma) (Figs. 26-1 through 26-4) Purpura is a condition characterized by the pooling of extravasated blood. The stimulating factor can be iatrogenic, factitial, or accidental trauma to vascular tissues contained within the dermis or submucosa. In circumstances where trauma is not involved, deficits in the platelets either quantitative or qualitative, clotting factors, or capillary fragility should be suspected. Initially purpura appear bright red, but tend to discolor with time, becoming purplish-blue and later brown-yellow. Because these lesions consist of extravascular blood, they do not blanch on pressure.

The three types of purpura – petechiae, ecchymoses, and hematoma are classified according to size and etiology. Petechiae are pinpoint nonraised circular red spots. The soft palate is the most common intraoral location for multifocal petechiae. Palatal petechiae may represent an early sign of infectious mononucleosis, scarlet fever, leukemia, bleeding diatheses, or blood dyscrasia. They may also indicate rupture of palatal capillaries due to coughing, sneezing, vomiting, or fellatio. Suction petechiae under a maxillary denture are not true purpura. They evolve as a result of candidal infection and the resulting inflammation of the orifices of accessory salivary glands, not because of denture-created negative pressure as previously believed.

An area of extravasated blood usually greater than 1cm in diameter is called an ecchymosis (common bruise). Careful physical evaluation may reveal the cause to be mechanical trauma, hemostatic disorders, Cushing's disease, neoplastic disease, primary idiopathic or secondary thrombocytopenic purpura, or use of anticoagulant drugs such as bishydroxycoumarin, warfarin, or heparin.

Hematomas are large pools of extravasated blood resulting from traumatic vascular severance. They occur most commonly in the oral cavity as a result of a blow to the face, tooth eruption, or rupture of the posterior superior alveolar vein during local anesthetic administration. They are usually dark red-brown or blue in color and tender to palpation. Purpura fade with time and require no specific treatment. Determining the underlying cause is the prime consideration.

Varicosity (Varix) (Fig. 26-5) A varix is a red-purple fluctuant swelling frequently seen in the elderly population. The swelling represents a venous dilation caused by reduced elasticity of the vascular wall as a result of aging, or by an internal blockage of the vein. The ventral surface of the anterior two thirds of the tongue is a frequent location. The lip and labial commissure are other common sites. Labial varices appear dark red to blue-purple. They are most commonly single, round, dome-shaped, and fluctuant. Palpation of the lesion will disperse the blood from the vessel, flattening the surface appearance; therefore the lesions are diascopy-positive.

Varices are benign and asymptomatic, and require no treatment. If they are of cosmetic concern to the patient, varices can be surgically removed without significant bleeding. Occasionally they are slightly firm because of fibrotic changes. Thrombosis is a rare complication. When multiple veins on the ventral tongue are prominent the condition is called phlebectasia linguae, or "caviar tongue."

Thrombus (Fig. 26-6) The series of events that includes trauma, activation of the clotting sequence, and formation of a blood clot typically results in the cessation of bleeding. Several days later clot breakdown occurs and normal blood flow resumes. In certain cases, if the clot does not dissolve, blood flow stagnates and a thrombus is formed.

Thrombi appear as raised red round nodules, typically in the labial mucosa. They are firm to palpation and may be slightly tender. No sexual predilection is evident, but thrombi are most commonly seen in patients over 30. Vascular plugs can concentrically enlarge to occlude the entire lumen of the vessel or mature and calcify to form a phlebolith. Phleboliths are rare oral findings that occur in the cheek, lips, or tongue. Radiographically they appear as doughnut-like, circular, radiopaque foci with a radiolucent center.

Hemangioma (Figs. 26-7 and 26-8) Hemangiomas are benign, enlarged, vascular hamartomas that may be seen in any soft-tissue intraoral location. They occur early in life and somewhat more commonly in females than in males. The dorsum of the tongue, gingiva, and buccal mucosa are common locations. Histologically they may be capillary or cavernous.

Hemangiomas, when situated deep within the connective tissue, do not alter the color of the mucosal surface. Superficial hemangiomas, in contrast, are red, blue, or purple in color, flat or slightly elevated, smooth-surfaced, and somewhat firm. Hemangiomas are positive to diascopy and may vary in size from a few millimeters to several centimeters. The borders are usually diffuse, and lobular surfaces are infrequent. Single hemangiomas are most common, whereas multiple tumors are seen in Maffucci's syndrome. Facial and oral hemangiomas form a component of Sturge-Weber syndrome.

Large soft tissue hemangiomas present management problems. Surgical excision, sclerosing agents, cryotherapy, and radiation therapy have been used to eliminate these lesions. A hemangioendothelioma is the malignant counterpart to the hemangioma, whereas Kaposi's sarcoma is another malignant vascular tumor seen in about 30% of AIDS patients.

RED LESIONS

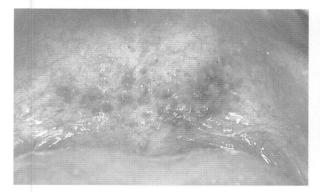

Fig. 26-1. Multiple red **petechiae** on the soft palate.

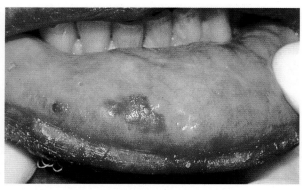

Fig. 26-2. Ecchymosis following lip trauma in a heparinized patient.

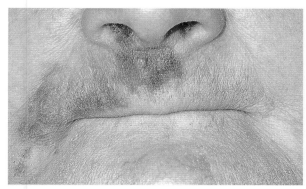

Fig. 26-3. Purplish-blue **hematoma** resulting from a blow to the face.

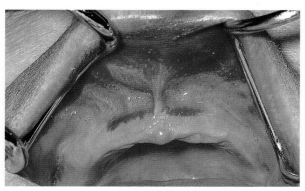

Fig. 26-4. Red intraoral **hematoma** of patient in Fig. 26-3.

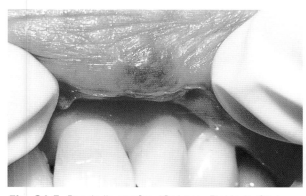

Fig. 26-5. Purple lip **varix.** (Courtesy Dr Linda Otis)

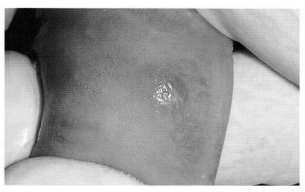

Fig. 26-6. Blue organizing **thrombus;** labial mucosa. (Courtesy Dr Ed Heslop)

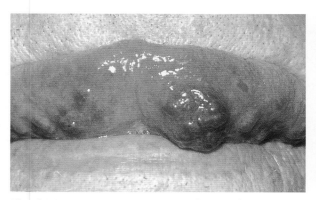

Fig. 26-7. Dome-shaped **hemangioma** of the ventral tongue. (Courtesy Dr Tom Razmus)

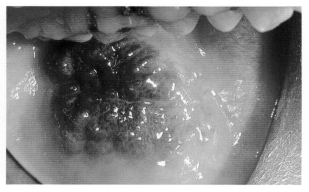

Fig. 26-8. Multinodular **hemangioma** of the buccal mucosa.

RED LESIONS

Hereditary Hemorrhagic Telangiectasia (Rendu-Osler-Weber) (Figs. 27-1 through 27-4) Hereditary hemorrhagic telangiectasia is a genetic disease that is inherited as an autosomal dominant trait. The disease is characterized by multiple telangiectasias, which are purplish red macules or slightly red papules representing permanently enlarged end-capillaries of the skin, mucosa, and other tissues. The lesions are usually 1 to 3 mm in size, lack central pulsation, and blanch upon diascopy. After puberty the size and number of lesions tend to increase with age. Males and females are affected equally. Bleeding is a prominent feature of this disease.

The lesions of hereditary hemorrhagic telangiectasia are located immediately subjacent to the mucosa and are easily traumatized, resulting in rupture, hemorrhage, and ulcer formation. Skin lesions are less subject to rupture because of the overlying cornified epithelium. The most common locations on the skin are the palms, fingers, nail beds, face, and neck. Mucosal lesions can be found on the lips, tongue, nasal septum, and conjunctivae. The gingiva and the hard palate are less commonly involved. Complications include epistaxis, gastrointestinal bleeding, melena, hematuria, cirrhosis, and pulmonary arteriovenous fistulae. Precautions are recommended with the use of inhalation analgesia, general anesthesia, oral surgical procedures, and hepatotoxic and anti-hemostatic drugs. Rupture of a telangiectasia may cause hemmorhage that is best controlled by pressure packs. History, clinical appearance, and histologic features are important in making the diagnosis.

Sturge-Weber Syndrome (Encephalotrigeminal Angiomatosis) (Figs. 27-5 through 27-8) Sturge-Weber syndrome is a rare congenital disorder that manifests venous angiomas of the leptomeninges of the brain, ipsilateral macular hemangiomas of the face, neuromuscular deficits, and oculo-oral lesions. The macular hemangioma of the facial skin, also termed "port-wine stain" or "nevus flammeus," is the most striking feature of the syndrome. The facial hemangioma is well-demarcated, flat or slightly raised, and red to purple in color. It blanches under pressure. It is present at birth, distributed along a branch of the trigeminal nerve, and typically extends to the patient's midline without crossing to the other side. The ophthalmic division of the trigeminal nerve is most frequently affected. No tenderness or inflammation is associated with the hemangioma, and it does not enlarge with age.

The altered venous blood flow caused by an angioma of the leptomeninges can result in cerebral cortical degeneration, seizures, mental retardation, and hemiplegia. On lateral skull radiographs gyriform calcifications characteristically appear as double-contoured "tram-lines." Approximately 30% of patients have ocular abnormalities including angiomas, colobomas, or glaucoma.

Vascular hyperplasia involving the buccal mucosa and lips is the most frequent oral finding. The palate, gingiva, and floor of the mouth may also be affected. Distribution of the bright red oral patches is to areas supplied by the branches of the trigeminal nerve. Like facial lesions, these patches stop abruptly at the midline. Involvement of the gingiva may produce edematous tissue and cause difficulty with hemostasis when surgical procedures involving these tissues are performed. Abnormal tooth eruption, macrocheilia, macrodontia, and macroglossia are sequelae of large vascular overgrowths. In areas of vascular hyperplasia oral surgery should be performed in accordance with strict hemostatic measures.

RED LESIONS

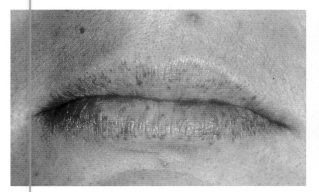

Fig. 27-1. Multiple lip telangiectasias; **hereditary hemorrhagic telangiectasia.**

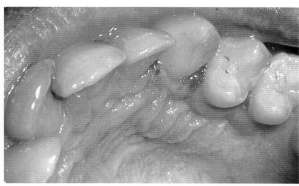

Fig. 27-2. Gingival telangiectasias; same patient as in Fig. 27-1 with **hereditary hemorrhagic telangiectasia.**

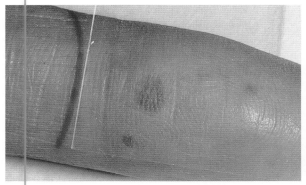

Fig. 27-3. Skin telangiectasias; **hereditary hemorrhagic telangiectasia.** (Courtesy Dr Margot van Dis)

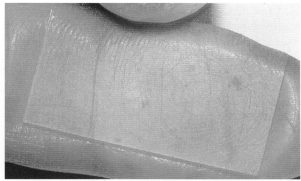

Fig. 27-4. Blanching of telangiectasias on diascopy; **hereditary hemorrhagic telangiectasia.** (Courtesy Dr Margot van Dis)

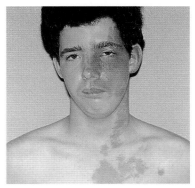

Fig. 27-5. Port-wine stain; **Sturge-Weber** syndrome. (Courtesy Dr Larry Skoczylas)

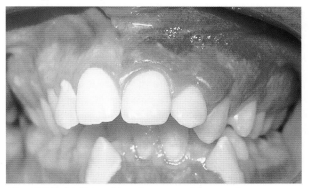

Fig. 27-6. Unilateral involvement of intraoral hemangioma; same patient as in Fig. 27-5 with **Sturge-Weber syndrome.** (Courtesy Dr Larry Skoczylas)

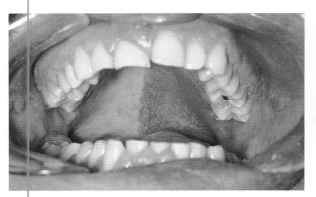

Fig. 27-7. Unilateral hemangioma of the palate; **Sturge-Weber syndrome.**

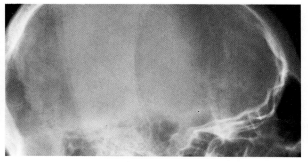

Fig. 27-8. Tram-line gyriform calcifications, lateral "skull radiograph"; same patient as in Fig. 27-7 with **Sturge-Weber syndrome.**

RED AND RED/WHITE LESIONS

Erythroplakia (Figs. 28-1 through 28-4) Erythroplakia is defined as a persistent velvety red patch that cannot be characterized clinically as any other condition. This term, like "leukoplakia," has no histologic connotation; however, the majority of erythroplakias are histologically diagnosed as epithelial dysplasia or worse, and thus have a much higher propensity for progression to carcinoma. Erythroplakias may be located anywhere in the mouth, but appear to be most prevalent in the mandibular mucobuccal fold, oropharynx and floor of the mouth. The redness of the lesion is a result of atrophic mucosa overlying a highly vascular submucosa. The border of the lesion is usually well-demarcated. There is no sexual predilection and patients over the age of 60 are most commonly affected.

Three clinical variants of erythroplakia have been recognized: (1) the homogenous form, which is completely red in appearance; (2) erythroleukoplakia, which has red patches interspersed with occasional leukoplakic areas; and (3) speckled erythroplakia, which contains white specks or granules scattered throughout the lesion. Biopsy is mandatory for all types of erythroplakia, because 91% of erythroplakias represent severe dysplasia, carcinoma in situ, or invasive squamous cell carcinoma. Close inspection of the entire oral cavity is also required, since 10 to 20% of these patients will have several erythroplakic areas, a phenomenon known as field cancerization.

Erythroleukoplakia and Speckled Erythroplakia (Fig. 28-5) Erythroleukoplakia and speckled erythroplakia, or "speckled leukoplakia," as some authors prefer, are precancerous red and white lesions. Erythroleukoplakia is a red patch with isolated leukoplakic areas, whereas speckled erythroplakia is a red patch that contains white speckles or granules throughout the entire lesion. A variant red-white lesion that has a nodular appearance is called proliferative verrucous leukoplakia.

Erythroleukoplakia and speckled erythroplakia have a male predilection, and most lesions are detected in patients over age 50. They may occur at any intraoral site, but frequently affect the lateral border of the tongue, buccal mucosa, and soft palate. These lesions are often associated with heavy smoking, alcoholism, and poor oral hygiene.

Fungal infections are common in speckled erythroplakias. *Candida albicans*, the predominant organism, has been isolated in the majority of cases; therefore the management of these lesions should include analysis for candida. The cause and effect relationship of candidiasis and speckled leukoplakia is unknown, but erythroplakia with leukoplakic regions confers a greater risk for atypical cytologic changes. Because of the increased risk for carcinoma, biopsy is mandatory of all red-white lesions.

Squamous Cell Carcinoma (Figs. 28-5 through 28-8) Squamous cell carcinoma is a malignant neoplasm of mucosal origin. It is the most common type of oral cancer, accounting for over 90% of all malignant neoplasms of the oral cavity. Oral cancer may occur at any age, but it is primarily a disease of the elderly; greater than 95% of oral cancers occur in persons over the age of 40. In the past, the prevalence was much higher in males, but the male to female ratio has dramatically decreased in recent years to approximately 2:1, owing to the increased number of women who smoke.

The exact cause of oral cancer is unknown. Cytologic atypism and mutagenesis may be a result of multiple factors associated with aging and exposure to a variety of biologic, chemical, and physical agents such as the following: infection with *Treponema pallidum*, herpes simplex virus, human papilloma virus, or *Candida albicans;* excessive use of tobacco and alcohol; nutritional deficiency states; oral neglect; chronic trauma; radiation; and immune suppression.

The most common site for intraoral squamous cell carcinoma is the lateral border and ventral surface of the tongue. Other intraoral sites, in descending order of involvement, are the oropharynx, floor of the mouth, gingiva, buccal mucosa, lip, and palate. The occurrence of squamous cell carcinoma of the lip has decreased dramatically in the past decade because of the increased use of protective sunscreening agents. The dorsal surface of the tongue is almost never affected.

The appearance of squamous cell carcinoma is highly variable, with over 90% of the cases having an erythroplakic component, and about 60% showing a leukoplakic component. A combination of colors and surface patterns, such as a red and white lesion that is exophytic, infiltrative, or ulcerated, indicates instability of the oral epithelium and is highly suggestive of carcinoma. Early lesions are often asymptomatic and slow-growing. As the lesion develops, the borders become diffuse and ragged, and induration and fixation ensue. If the mucosal surface becomes ulcerated, the most frequent oral complaint is that of a persistent "sore" or "irritation." Not uncommonly, patients may complain of numbness or a burning sensation, swelling, or difficulty in speaking or swallowing. Extension of lesions to several centimeters in diameter can result if treatment is delayed, permitting large lesions to invade and destroy vital osseous structures.

Spread of squamous cell carcinoma occurs by local extension, or by way of the lymphatic vessels. Staging of the tumor according to size (T), regional lymph nodes (N), and distant metastases (M) affords assessment of the extent of disease. Surgery and radiation therapy have been the principal forms of treatment for oral cancer.

The prognosis for oral cancer depends, in large measure, on the site involved, the clinical stage at the time of diagnosis, the width of the tumor at its greatest diameter, the patient's access to adequate health care, ability to cope and mount an immunologic response. Early treatment is paramount; therefore biopsy should be initiated if there is suspicion of neoplasia.

RED AND RED/WHITE LESIONS

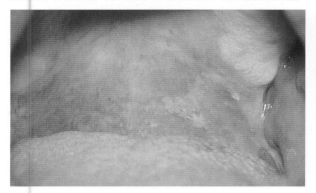

Fig. 28-1. Erythroplakia not discernible until the tongue is depressed as seen in Fig. 28-2.

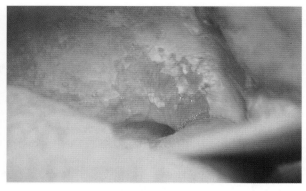

Fig. 28-2. Erythroplakia with leukoplakic border; biopsy revealed epithelial dysplasia.

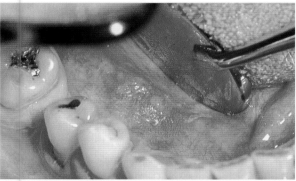

Fig. 28-3. Erythroplakia along the sublingual caruncle; biopsy revealed carcinoma in situ. (Courtesy Dr Robert Craig)

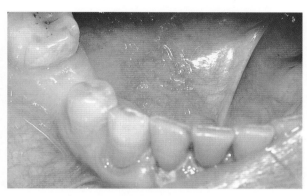

Fig. 28-4. Erythroplakia of the floor of the mouth; biopsy revealed squamous cell carcinoma.

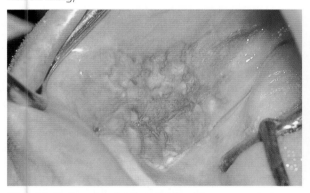

Fig. 28-5. Erythroleukoplakia; biopsy revealed squamous cell carcinoma.

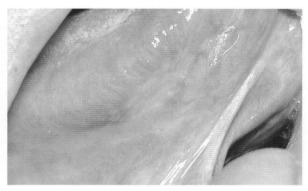

Fig. 28-6. Squamous cell carcinoma of the tongue adjacent to area seen in Fig. 28-5; example of **field cancerization.**

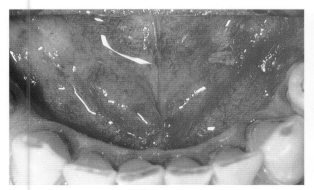

Fig. 28-7. Subtle **erythroleukoplakia** that proved to be squamous cell carcinoma. (Courtesy Dr Robert Craig)

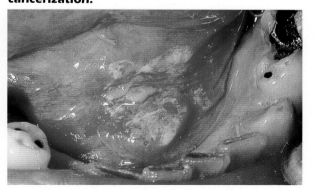

Fig. 28-8. Speckled erythroplakia; biopsy revealed squamous cell carcinoma. (Courtesy Dr Robert Craig)

RED AND RED/WHITE LESIONS

Lichen Planus (Figs. 29-1 through 29-6) Lichen planus is a common skin disease that frequently has mucosal manifestations. The etiology and pathogenesis are unknown, although evidence suggests that lichen planus is an immunologic disorder, possibly an autoimmune disease, in which T-lymphocytes destroy the basal cell layer of the affected epithelium. Both CD4 and CD8 T-cell subsets have been identified in the submucosal lymphocyte population. Nervous and high-strung persons are predisposed to lichen planus. The majority of patients are females over the age of 40. The disease exhibits a protracted course with periods of remission and exacerbation.

The skin lesions of lichen planus initially consist of small, flat-topped, red papules with a depressed central area. The lesions may enlarge and become polygonal in shape or coalesce into larger plaques. The papules progressively acquire a violaceous hue and surface lichenification, which consists of fine white striae. The lesions usually itch and may change color to yellow or brown before resolution. Bilateral distribution on the flexor surfaces of the extremities is common, occasionally involving the fingernails. Patients with characteristic purple, polygonal, pruritic papules on the skin often have concurrent intraoral lesions.

Oral lesions of lichen planus may have one of four appearances: atrophic, erosive, striated (reticular), or plaquelike. More than one form may affect a single patient. The most frequently affected site is the buccal mucosa. The tongue, lips, palate, gingiva, and floor of the mouth may also be affected. Bilateral and relatively symmetrical lesions are common. Patients with reticular oral lichen planus characteristically have multiple delicate white lines or papules arranged in a lacy, web-like network known as "striae of Wickham." The glistening white areas are often asymptomatic but of cosmetic concern. They may involve large areas.

Atrophic lichen planus results from atrophy of the epithelium and predominantly appears as a red, non-ulcerated mucosal patch. Wickham's striae are often present at the border of the lesion. When the attached gingiva is affected, the term "desquamative gingivitis" has been used.

Erosive lichen planus occurs if the surface epithelium is completely lost and ulceration results. The buccal mucosa and tongue are commonly affected sites. Initially, a vesicle or bulla may appear which eventually erodes producing ulceration. Mature lesions have irregular red borders, a yellowish necrotic central pseudomembrane, and an annular white patch often at the periphery. The condition is intermittently painful and may onset rapidly. All of these features are helpful in differentiating oral lichen planus from other clinically similar-appearing lesions such as leukoplakia, erythroplakia, candidiasis, lupus erythematosus, pemphigoid, and erythema multiforme.

The least common type of lichen planus is the asymptomatic plaque form. This lesion is a solid white plaque or patch that has a smooth to slightly irregular surface and an asymmetric configuration. Lesions are commonly found on buccal or glossal mucosa. Patients may be unaware of these lesions.

In many cases clinical appearance alone can confirm the diagnosis of oral lichen planus, and a biopsy is not necessary. Asymptomatic intraoral lesions can be left alone. Biopsy of the atrophic or erosive form should be performed at the border of the lesion.

The oral lesions of lichen planus tend to be more persistent than those of the skin. A vacation, change in routine, or discharge of psychologically burdensome problems can bring about abrupt and dramatic resolution of the lesions. Chronic, symptomatic, erosive lichen planus lesions are best managed with topical or systemic steroids and immunosuppressants. A small number of patients with oral lichen planus are diabetic and should be tested for glucose intolerance. Carcinomatous transformation has been reported (in less than 100 cases) to have an association with erosive lichen planus and tobacco use. The true cause and effect relationship, however, has yet to be established for squamous cell carcinoma and lichen planus.

Electrogalvanic White Lesion (Figs. 29-7 and 29-8) Electrogalvanic white lesions closely resemble the hypertrophic form of lichen planus. This disorder is more apparent after the age of 30 and frequently occurs on the buccal mucosa, immediately adjacent to a metallic restoration. Mild cases are asymptomatic, whereas erosive cases can cause a burning type of pain. Histologically this lesion mimics lichen planus. Electric microcurrents induced by dissimilar restorations is one explanation for this phenomenon. Interestingly, lichenoid drug reactions, which are similar in appearance to electrogalvanic white lesions, can be caused by the systemic application of the same metals (mercury and gold) found in dental restorations. Treatment consists of replacing the restoration with a different restorative material, preferably gold, porcelain, glass ionomer, or composite materials. The prognosis is excellent.

RED AND RED/WHITE LESIONS

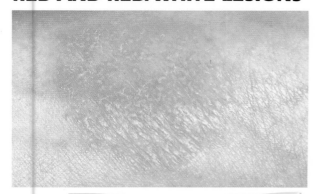

Fig. 29-1. Violaceous skin plaque with lichenification on forearm indicative of **lichen planus.**

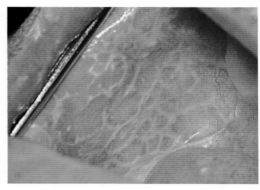

Fig. 29-2. Characteristic Wickham striae of **reticular lichen planus.** (Courtesy Dr Birgit Glass)

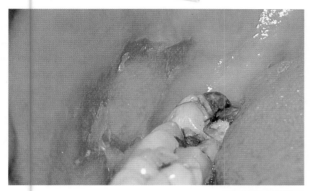

Fig. 29-3. Painful denuded patches of **erosive lichen planus.**

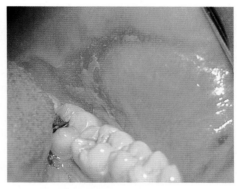

Fig. 29-4. Erosive lichen planus; same patient as in Fig 29-3.

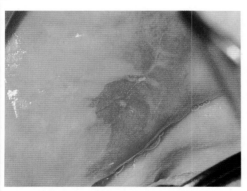

Fig. 29-5. Red atrophic lichen planus on buccal mucosa after biopsy. (Courtesy Dr Tom Razmus)

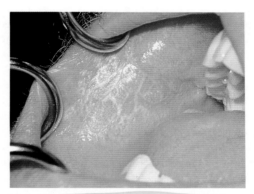

Fig. 29-6. Plaque form of lichen planus with a few striae.

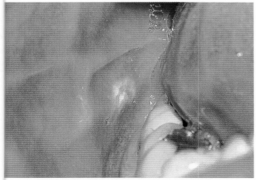

Fig. 29-7. Electrogalvanic white lesion that has a configuration coincident to the adjacent class-V alloy restoration.

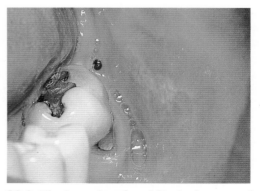

Fig. 29-8. Electrogalvanic white lesion opposite side in the same patient as seen in Fig. 29-7.

RED AND RED/WHITE LESIONS

Lupus Erythematosus (Figs. 30-1 through 30-4)

Lupus erythematosus (LE) exists in three forms: chronic discoid lupus erythematosus (CDLE), which only involves the skin; systemic lupus erythematosus (SLE), in which multiple organ systems are involved; and subacute cutaneous lupus erythematosus, a cutaneous variant with mild systemic symptoms. The cause of all three types is unknown.

CDLE, the benign form of the disease, is a purely mucocutaneous disorder. It may appear at any age, but predominates in females over the age of 40. CDLE is classically characterized by a red butterfly rash symmetrically distributed across the bridge of the nose. Other prominent photosensitive areas of the face, including the cheeks, malar areas, forehead, scalp, and ears, may be involved.

The lesions of LE are chronic with periods of exacerbation and remission. Mature lesions exhibit three zones: an atrophic center lined by a hyperkeratotic middle zone which is surrounded by an erythematous periphery. Frequently there is hypopigmentation of the lesion resulting from melanocytic damage at the epidermal-dermal junction. Telangiectasias, blackheads, and a fine scale are common dermal findings. The lesions are usually limited to the upper portion of the body, particularly the head and neck.

Twenty to 40% of patients with LE have oral lesions. These lesions may develop before or after skin lesions develop. Lip lesions are red with a white to silvery, scaly margin. A sun-exposed lower lip at the vermilion border is a common site, whereas the upper lip is usually involved as a result of direct extension of dermal lesions. Intraoral lesions are frequently diffuse and erythematous, with ulcerative and white components.

Occasionally CDLE appears as isolated white plaques. The buccal mucosa is the most frequent intraoral site, followed by the tongue, palate and gingiva. Alternating parallel red and white lines in a radial arrangement are an important diagnostic feature, along with the appearance of multiple lesions on several surfaces. These lesions may mimic lichen planus; however, concurrent ear involvement helps to exclude the diagnosis of lichen planus. Ulcerative lesions are painful and require treatment. Avoidance of emotional stress, cold, sunlight, and hot spicy foods is necessary. The use of sunscreens, topical steroids, systemic steroids, and antimalarial agents have proven effective. Patients using antimalarial agents require close ophthalmologic followup.

SLE, an autoimmune collagen disease, is characterized by the production of antinuclear and anti-DNA antibodies that participate in immunologically mediated tissue injury.

Patients often complain of fatigue, fever, and joint pain. Generalized nontender lymphadenopathy is often present. Hepatomegaly, splenomegaly, peripheral neuropathy, and hematologic abnormalities may also be seen. Strict avoidance of sun exposure is necessary, since sunburn can trigger acute reactions. Involvement of the kidneys and heart is a common occurrence that may prove fatal. Skin and oral lesions may accompany SLE, but there is little chance of conversion from discoid to systemic lupus. Patients with SLE often suffer concurrently from other autoimmune collagen-vascular diseases such as Sjögren's syndrome and rheumatoid arthritis. Allergic mucositis, candidiasis, leukoplakia, erythroleukoplakia, and lichen planus must be considered in the differential diagnosis of oral LE lesions. Biopsy and histologic examination with immunofluorescence confirms the diagnosis. Precautions are advised in the dental treatment of patients with lupus erythematosus who may be taking high doses of systemic steroids, because of their predisposition to delayed wound healing, the risk of infection, and the possibility of stress-induced adrenal crisis characterized by cardiovascular collapse. These patients are also at risk for cardiomyopathy which requires antibiotic prophylaxis.

Lichenoid and Lupus-like Drug Eruption (Figs. 30-5 through 30-8)

Reticular or erosive lesions similar in appearance to lichen planus and lupus erythematosus may occur in association with a variety of systemic medications. Although the appearance may be quite varied, white linear plaques with red margins are common. The lesions may erupt upon immediate or after prolonged use of a drug. Persistent inflammatory changes may result in large erythematous areas, eventual mucosal ulceration, and pain. Drug-induced lupus erythematosus is often associated with arthritis, fever, and renal disease. Hydralazine and procainamide are the most common instigators of lupus-like drug eruptions. Other drugs known to cause lupus-like eruptions include gold, griseofulvin, isoniazid, methyldopa, penicillin, phenytoin, procainamide, streptomycin, and trimethadione. Drugs known to induce lichenoid eruptions include the following: chloroquine, dapsone, furosemide, gold, mercury, methyldopa, palladium, penicillamine, phenothiazines, quinidine, thiazides, certain antibiotics, and heavy metals. Consultation with a physician and withdrawal of the offending medication will lead to regression of the lesion. A substitute drug is usually selected to manage the patient's systemic problem.

RED AND RED/WHITE LESIONS

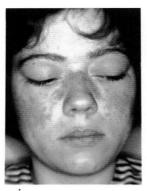

Fig. 30-1. Butterfly rash; **chronic discoid lupus erythematosus.**

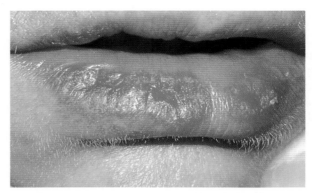

Fig. 30-2. Red scaly lip lesion of **chronic discoid lupus erythematosus**. (Courtesy Dr James Cottone)

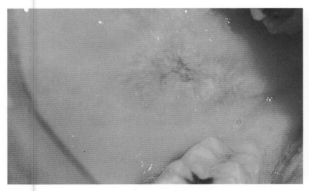

Fig. 30-3. Alternating radial red and white lines; **chronic discoid lupus erythematosus.**

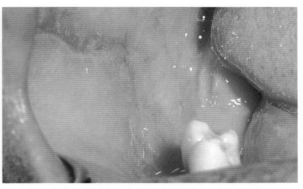

Fig. 30-4. Red and white curvilinear plaque; **chronic discoid lupus erythematosus.** (Courtesy Dr James Cottone)

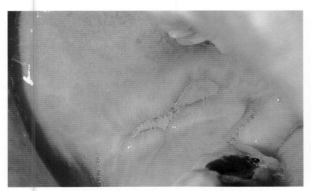

Fig. 30-5. Lupus-like drug eruption following the administration of amitriptyline.

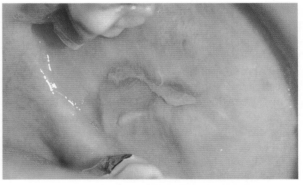

Fig. 30-6. Ulcerated **lupus-like drug eruption** opposite buccal mucosa, same patient as in Fig. 30-5.

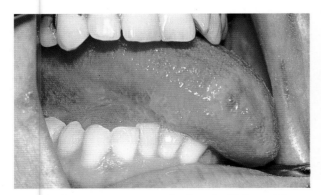

Fig. 30-7. White plaques and striae of a **lichenoid drug eruption** subsequent to furosemide therapy.

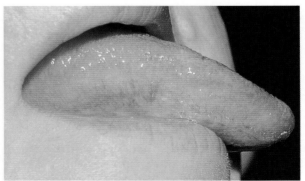

Fig. 30-8. Withdrawal of furosemide resulted in complete resolution of **lichenoid drug eruption** seen in Fig. 30-7.

RED AND RED/WHITE LESIONS

Acute Pseudomembranous Candidiasis (Thrush) (Figs. 31-1 and 31-2) Acute pseudomembranous candidiasis, an opportunistic infection, is caused by an overgrowth of the superficial fungus *Candida albicans*. It appears as diffuse, curdy, or velvety white mucosal plaques that can be wiped off, leaving a red, raw, or bleeding surface. The organism is a common inhabitant of the oral cavity, gastrointestinal tract, and vagina. Infants whose mothers display vaginal thrush at the time of birth and adults who have experienced an upset in the normal oral microflora due to antibiotics, steroids, or systemic alterations such as diabetes, hypoparathyroidism, immunodeficiency, or chemotherapy are frequently affected. There is no racial or sexual predilection.

Acute pseudomembranous candidiasis is usually found on the buccal mucosa, tongue, and soft palate. Clinically the white plaques appear in clusters that have an erythematous border. A peculiar pattern is seen in asthmatic patients who use a steroid inhaler. The pattern appears as a circular or oval reddish-white patch at the site of aerosol contact on the palate. Diagnosis can be made by clinical examination, fungal culture, or direct microscopic examination of tissue scrapings. A potassium hydroxide (KOH), Gram's, or periodic acid-Schiff (PAS)-stained cytologic smear will reveal budding organisms with branching pseudohyphae. Topical application of antifungal medication for 2 weeks usually produces resolution.

Chronic Keratotic Candidiasis (Hyperplastic) (Figs. 31-3 and 31-4) Chronic keratotic candidiasis is caused by organisms of the candida sp. that penetrate the mucosal surface and stimulate a hyperplastic response. Chronic irritation, poor oral hygiene, and xerostomia are predisposing factors; thus smokers and denture wearers are commonly affected. Chiefly involved is the dorsum of the tongue, palate, and labial commissures. The lesion invariably has a distinctive raised border and a white, pebbly surface with an occasional red area; thus the condition may resemble leukoplakia or erythroleukoplakia. The scattered erythematous components are a result of mucosal cell layer destruction.

The white patch of chronic keratotic candidiasis cannot be peeled off, requiring the diagnosis to be made by biopsy. Microscopically the organisms may be identified by routine hematoxylin and eosin stain or, more appropriately, by the PAS stain. With adequate topical application of an anti-fungal agent, resolution usually occurs. In some instances surgical stripping may be required. All patients with chronic keratotic candidiasis should be followed closely, since this form may be related to speckled erythroplakia, a lesion which is often premalignant or worse.

Acute Atrophic Candidiasis (Antibiotic Sore Mouth) (Fig. 31-5) The use of broad spectrum antibiotics, particularly tetracyclines, can result in the oral condition termed "acute atrophic candidiasis." This fungal infection is the result of an imbalance in the oral ecosystem between *Lactobacillus acidophilus* and *Candida albicans*. Antibiotics taken by the patient reduce the *Lactobacillus* population and permit candidal organisms to flourish. The infection produces desquamated areas of surface mucosa that appear as diffuse, nonelevated red patches. Burning pain is the most frequent chief complaint. The distribution of the patches of acute atrophic candidiasis is sometimes indicative of the cause. Lesions affecting the buccal mucosa, lips, and oropharynx often suggest the systemic administration of antibiotics, whereas redness of the tongue and palate are more common following the use of antibiotic troches. When the tongue is affected a surface devoid of filiform papillae is common. It is rare for candidiasis to affect the attached gingiva; if this is the clinical finding, then severe immune suppression is a distinct possibility. The diagnosis of a candidal infection should be confirmed by demonstration of budding organisms or hyphal forms on a stained cytologic smear. Treatment is with antifungal agents.

Angular Cheilitis (Fig. 31-6) Angular cheilitis is a chronic painful condition involving the labial commissures caused by *Candida albicans*. Clinically, angular cheilitis appears red and fissured, with the periphery of the lesion less erythematous than central areas. Crusting and brownish granulomatous nodules may be concurrent. Discomfort caused by opening the mouth may limit normal oral function. Predisposing factors and treatment have been previously discussed.

Chronic Atrophic Candidiasis (Denture Stomatitis) (Figs. 31-7 and 31-8) Chronic atrophic candidiasis is the most common form of chronic candidiasis. It is present in 15 to 65% of complete and partial denture wearers, particularly elderly females who wear their dentures at night; rarely dentate patients may also be affected. The mandible, however, is rarely involved. Misnomers for this disease are the terms "denture sore mouth" and "denture base allergy".

Chronic atrophic candidiasis is caused by candidal organisms located under the denture base. There are three stages of mucosal alterations. The earliest lesions are red pinpoint areas of hyperemia limited to the orifices of the palatal minor salivary glands. Progression produces a diffuse erythema of the hard palate that is sometimes accompanied by epithelial desquamation. Papillary hyperplasia is the third stage. It may be generalized or restricted to relief areas. Rarely a fourth stage is apparent; the enlargement of palatal papules to form red nodules on the vault of the palate. Effective therapy requires antifungal treatment of the mucosa and denture base. The role of trauma, such as the rocking action of the denture, may perpetuate the condition.

RED AND RED/WHITE LESIONS

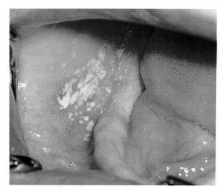

Fig. 31-1. Thrush in an immunosuppressed patient. (Courtesy Dr Sol Silverman)

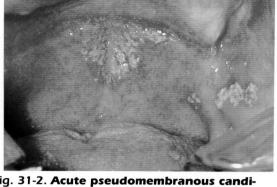

Fig. 31-2. Acute pseudomembranous candidiasis in a patient that uses a steroid inhaler. (Courtesy Dr Geza Terezhalmy)

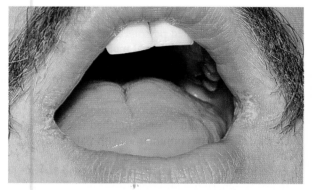

Fig. 31-3. Chronic hyperplastic candidiasis at the labial commissure which extends onto the buccal mucosa.

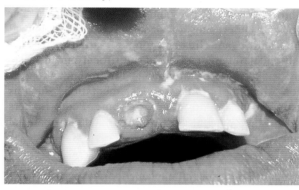

Fig. 31-4. White keratotic plaques of **hyperplastic candidiasis** in a debiliated patient.

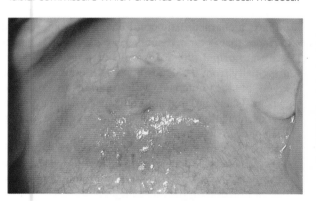

Fig. 31-5. Acute atrophic candidiasis limited to non-denture-bearing area, due to steroid inhalant.

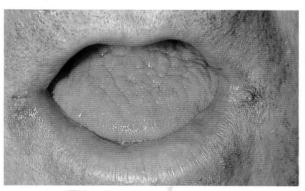

Fig. 31-6. Angular cheilitis. (Courtesy Dr James Cottone)

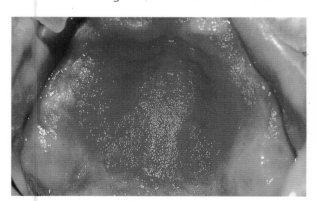

Fig. 31-7. Papillary hyperplasia; the third stage of denture stomatitis. (Courtesy Dr Ken Abramovitch)

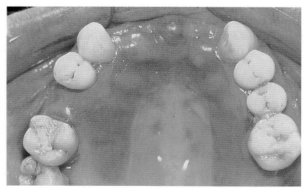

Fig. 31-8. Chronic atrophic candidiasis limited to partial denture bearing area. (Courtesy Dr Nancy Mantich)

Intraoral Findings by Surface Change

NODULES

Retrocuspid Papilla (Figs. 35-1 and 35-2) This anatomic structure is not seen in all individuals. It consists of a firm, round, fibro-epithelial papule, usually 1 to 4 mm in diameter, located on the attached gingiva lingual to the mandibular cuspids just below or several millimeters below the marginal gingiva. The surface mucosa is usually pink, soft, and smooth. Rarely the lesions may be pedunculated and the stalk can be lifted off the gingiva by a periodontal probe. This condition is a variation of normal and is frequently found bilaterally. Some authorities state that the retrocuspid papilla is a developmental anomaly that represents a variant form of fibroma. Apparently the retrocuspid papilla is present in most children, but regresses with maturity; thus the incidence and size decrease with increasing age. The retrocuspid papilla has no sexual predilection, and no treatment is necessary unless interference with a removable prosthesis is anticipated.

Lymphoepithelial Cyst (Figs. 35-3 and 35-4) The lymphoepithelial cyst is an encapsulated, fluid-filled dermal or submucosal mass that arises from epithelium entrapped in lymphoid tissue that has undergone cystic transformation. It is usually asymptomatic, but may enlarge and spontaneously fistulate. Most appear in children and young adults. No sexual predilection has been demonstrated.

When the lymphoepithelial cyst is derived from degenerative tissue of the second branchial arch, it is referred to as a branchial cleft cyst, and it appears on the lateral aspect of the neck just anterior and deep to the superior third of the sternocleidomastoid muscle near the angle of the mandible. Occasionally the cyst may occur in the proximity of the parotid gland. The extraoral lymphoepithelial cyst is a well-circumscribed, soft, fluctuant mass that is rubbery to the touch.

Common sites for the intraoral lymphoepithelial cyst are the floor of the mouth, lingual frenum, ventral tongue, and base of the tongue. These small swellings, rarely exceeding 1 cm in diameter, are characteristically well-circumscribed, soft, and doughy, with a yellow color. Palpation yields a slightly moveable nodule. When located in the anterior floor, the lesion may resemble a mucous retention cyst. Infrequently, multiple lymphoepithelial cysts can be found.

Histologically, lymphoepithelial cysts are usually lined with stratified squamous epithelium, but occasionally pseudostratified, columnar, or cuboidal epithelium is found. A fibrous connective tissue wall surrounds the lesion, which contains dark-staining lymphoid aggregates with prominent germinal centers. The luminal fluid is yellow and viscous. Excisional biopsy should be performed to provide histologic confirmation. Recurrence of the lymphoepithelial cyst is rare.

Torus, Exostosis, and Osteoma (Figs. 35-5 through 35-8) Tori, exostoses, and peripheral osteomas are readily recognizable bony hard nodules that appear histologically identical. The term used depends on location, appearance, and systemic associations.

Bony protuberances of the jaws, localized to the palatal midline or mandibular lingual attached gingiva, are termed "tori". They are the most common intraoral lesions that are exophytic by nature. Females are most frequently affected. Tori have smooth rounded contours, normal-appearing or slightly pale mucosa, and a sessile base. Often tori are found to have a lobulated surface. Internally they are composed of cortical bone with occasional areas of spongy bone.

Bony outgrowths in alternate locations are termed "exostoses". The facial aspect of the maxillary and mandibular alveolar ridge are common sites. Infrequently the palatal alveolar ridge adjacent to maxillary molars is affected. Usually exostoses are multiple hard nodules that demonstrate crease-like folds between distinct nodules. The surface mucosa is firm, taut, and white to pale pink.

Tori and exostoses tend to increase slowly in size with increasing age, but remain asymptomatic unless traumatized. Following a traumatic incident, patients may be concerned about neoplasia and insist that the bony mass is enlarging or that it was not present prior to the injury. Removal is generally unnecessary unless prompted by cosmetic, prosthodontic, psychological, or traumatic considerations.

Osteomas are considered to be neoplastic growths that are distinct from the developmental lesions, tori and exostoses, because osteomas have more growth potential, tend to be larger, and may be confined to soft tissue. Patients with osteomas should be examined radiographically for multiple impacted supernumerary teeth, which may indicate the presence of Gardner's syndrome (see p.14). This autosomal dominant condition is characterized by osteomas, dermal cysts, multiple impacted and supernumerary teeth, and intestinal polyposis with a high propensity for malignant transformation. The majority of patients with Gardner's syndrome will demonstrate malignant polyposis by age 40; therefore all patients with this condition require close medical management.

NODULES

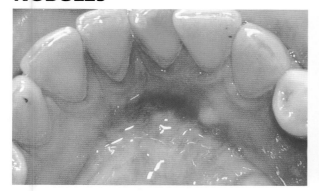

Fig. 35-1. **Retrocuspid papilla** appearing as a pink papule.

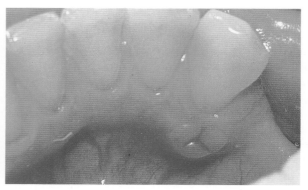

Fig. 35-2. Unusual clefting of a **retrocuspid papilla.**

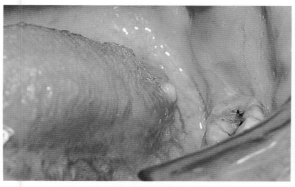

Fig. 35-3. Yellow **lymphoepithelial cyst** on the margin of the tongue.

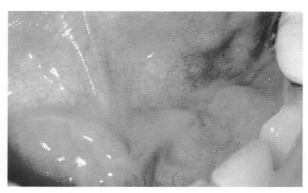

Fig. 35-4. Pinkish nodule in the floor of the mouth representing a **lymphoepithelial cyst.**

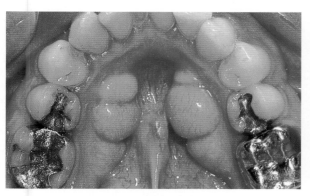

Fig. 35-5. Extensive **mandibular tori.**

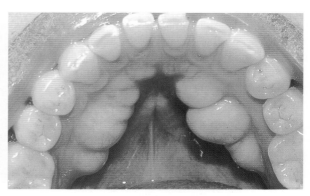

Fig. 35-6. Multinodular **mandibular tori.**

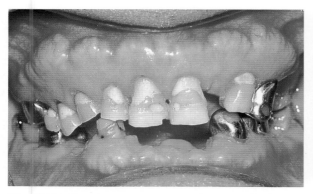

Fig. 35-7. **Exostoses** apparent at the mucogingival junction of the maxilla and mandible.

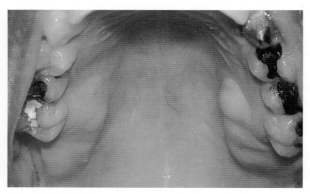

Fig. 35-8. Palatal **exostoses.** (Courtesy Dr Tom McDavid)

NODULES

Irritation Fibroma and Peripheral Odontogenic Fibroma (Figs. 36-1 and 36-2) The irritation fibroma is one of the most common benign lesions of the oral cavity. It results from reactive hyperplasia caused by a chronic irritant; thus this lesion is not a true neoplasm as the term "fibroma" seems to imply. True neoplastic fibromas are a rare intraoral finding.

Typically the irritation fibroma appears as a well-defined, pale-pink, slow-growing papule that with time enlarges to form a nodule. This smooth and symmetrically round lesion is firm and painless to palpation. Infrequently a leukoplakic, roughened, or ulcerated surface is present. The base is usually sessile. This growth can arise on any soft tissue location in the mouth, including buccal mucosa, labial mucosa, gingiva, or tongue. Histologically an interlacing mass of dense collagenous tissue is found subjacent to thinned epithelium. Fibromas are best treated by removing the source of the irritation together with surgical excision. Fibromas recur infrequently if treated properly. Multiple intraoral fibromas may be associated with the condition tuberous sclerosis (Bourneville-Pringle's disease), which is characterized by seizures, mental deficiency, and sebaceous adenomas that are in fact fibromas.

The peripheral odontogenic fibroma is clinically similar to the irritation fibroma, but is characterized by its unique location and tissue of origin. In most cases the peripheral fibroma is found as a circumscribed swelling in the region of the interdental papilla, generally located anterior to the molar teeth. A cup-like erosion of the underlying alveolar bone may be radiographically evident. It probably arises from cellular components of the periodontal ligament. Microscopically, clusters of odontogenic epithelium among dense collagenous tissue is found.

Lipoma (Figs. 36-3 and 36-4) The lipoma is a common dermal tumor, but a rare intraoral finding. This benign neoplasm is composed of mature fat cells surrounded by a thin, fibrous connective tissue wall. Adults over the age of 30 years are commonly affected, and no sexual predilection exists. Intraorally the lipoma appears as a well-circumscribed, smooth-surfaced, dome-shaped or diffusely elevated nodule that is yellow to pale pink in color. Occasionally lipomas may be polypoid, pedunculated, or lobulated.

Lipomas are slow-growing submucosal nodules that occur on the buccal mucosa, tongue, floor of the mouth, alveolar fold, and lip. The palate is a rare site of involvement. Palpation reveals a soft, movable, and compressible submucosal mass that has a slightly doughy consistency. Therapy consists of surgical removal, which includes the base of the lesion. Lipomas rarely recur.

Lipofibroma (Fig. 36-5) The lipofibroma is a rare benign intraoral neoplasm of mixed connective tissue origin. Microscopically it is a well-demarcated submucosal mass that consists of mature lipid-containing cells with a significant fibrous connective tissue component. Clinically the appearance is a blend of a fibroma and lipoma. It is generally found on labial and buccal mucosa. On palpation the lesion is non-indurated, movable, painless, and soft or firm depending on the lipoid-to-collagen content. These lesions are slow growing, but if left untreated they can grow to several centimeters in diameter.

Traumatic Neuroma (Amputation Neuroma) (Fig. 36-6) The traumatic neuroma results from a hyperplastic response to nerve damage following severance of a large nerve fiber. Intraorally the traumatic neuroma is frequently encountered in the mandibular mucobuccal fold in the region adjacent to the mental foramen. Other locations include the area facial to the mandibular incisors, the area lingual to the retromolar pad, and the ventral tongue. Size of the lesion depends upon both the degree of insult and degree of hyperplastic response.

Traumatic neuromas are usually very small nodules, measuring less than 0.5 cm in diameter. Visualization may be difficult if the lesion is located deep below normal oral mucosa. Neuromas are painful when palpated. Pressure applied to the neuroma elicits a response often described as an "electric shock." Multiple neuromas discovered on lips, tongue, or palate may indicate the possibility of multiple endocrine neoplasia Type IIb. Treatment of the traumatic neuroma is surgical excison or intralesional injection with corticosteroids. Excision may further damage the nerve and lead to recurrence.

Neurofibroma (Figs. 36-7 and 36-8) Neoplastic proliferation of all the elements of a peripheral nerve, including the sheath of Schwann, results in the benign tumor neurofibroma. They most commonly appear as firm pink nodules. Clinically neurofibromas may be solitary, diffuse, or over 1000 in number. Solitary nodules are rare. More commonly, multiple large neurofibromas are encountered, which are associated with neurofibromatosis (von Recklinghausen's disease).

Neurofibromatosis is an autosomal dominant disorder characterized by skin pigmentations (café-au-lait spots and axillary freckling) and multiple neurofibromas apparent in the skin, oral cavity, bone, and gastrointestinal tract. A pathognomonic sign of this disorder is Crowe's sign, which consists of more than 5 café-au-lait spots and axillary freckling.

Intraoral neurofibromas may be located on the dental arches, buccal mucosa, tongue, and lips. Most soft tissue neurofibromas are asymptomatic; however, those arising within deeper tissues may produce pain and paresthesia. Diffuse neurofibromas are striking for their firmness and irregular nodular surface that often results in physical deformity. In some cases neurofibromas undergo sarcomatous change, necessitating close followup. Solitary neurofibromas not associated with von Recklinghausen's disease have no tendency for malignant transformation.

NODULES

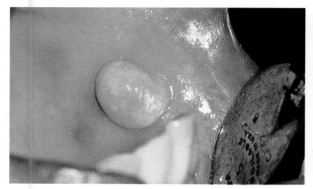

Fig. 36-1. Large nodule; **irritation fibroma.**

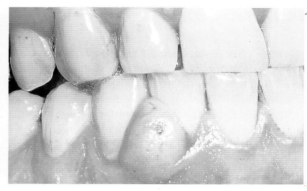

Fig. 36-2. Pink interdental papule; **peripheral odontogenic fibroma.**

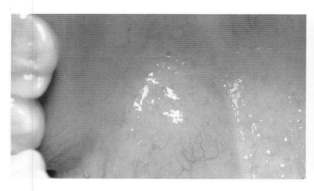

Fig. 36-3. Lipoma arising at the junction of the hard and soft palate. (Courtesy Dr Dale Miles)

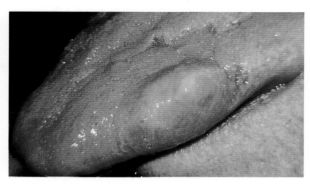

Fig. 36-4. Diffuse **lipoma** of the lateral margin of the tongue.

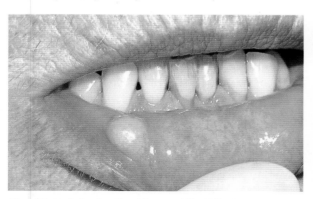

Fig. 36-5. Raised yellowish mass; **lipofibroma.** (Courtesy Dr Birgit Glass)

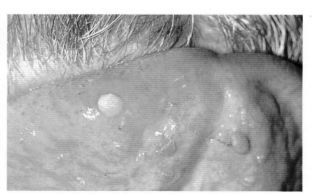

Fig. 36-6. Pink **traumatic neuroma** (near midline) and a whitish papilloma. (Courtesy Dr Jerry Cioffi)

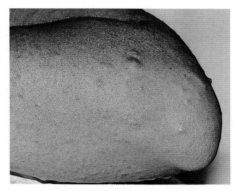

Fig. 36-7. Café-au-lait spots and **neurofibromas;** von Recklinghausen's disease.

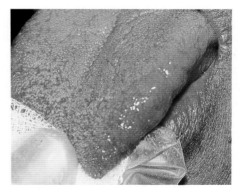

Fig. 36-8. Neurofibroma of the lateral margin of the tongue.

PAPULONODULES

Papilloma (Squamous Papilloma) (Figs. 37-1 and 37-2) Papillomas are the most common benign epithelial neoplasm of the oral cavity. They appear as small, pink-white, exophytic masses that are usually less than 1 cm in diameter. The surface of the papule may be smooth, pink, and pebbly, or have numerous small finger-like projections. The base is pedunculated and well-circumscribed. Intraoral lesions are typically soft, whereas those on exposed areas of the lips are usually rough and scaly. Solitary lesions are the general finding, but multiple lesions are occasionally seen. A viral etiology is probable with a recent study implicating human papilloma virus (HPV) Types 6 and 11 in 35% of the squamous papillomas examined. Because the papilloma is slow growing, any rapidly advancing papillomatous lesion should be suspected to be a more aggressive lesion.

The mean age of occurrence of the papilloma is 35 years and more cases have been documented in males than in females. The most common location is the uvulo-palatal complex, followed by the tongue and frenum, lips, buccal mucosa, and gingiva. Other HPV-induced lesions such as the condyloma acuminatum, focal epithelial hyperplasia (Heck's disease), and verruca vulgaris share similar clinical features, but are microscopically distinct. Treatment is complete excision, including the base. Recurrence is rare. There have been no documented cases of malignant transformation.

Verruca Vulgaris (Figs. 37-3 and 37-4) Verruca vulgaris is a common skin growth that seldom occurs intraorally. The etiologic agent is a papilloma virus. Virally induced cellular changes result in the characteristic clinical findings. Typically the lesional surface is rough and raised with white finger-like projections. The whiteness of intraoral verrucae varies depending on the amount of surface keratinization. Pink areas are not unusual at the lesional base.

Verrucae are commonly located on the skin, vermilion border, labial and buccal mucosa, tongue, and attached gingiva. The base of the lesion is broad, but the size is usually less than 1 cm. Clinically a verruca may appear identical to a papilloma, although the clefts are more shallow and the mass more sessile. Viral inclusion bodies are frequently seen histologically. Individuals with skin verrucae are more likely to have oral lesions as a result of autoinoculation. Occasionally a lesion may regress spontaneously. If not, treatment is complete excision or ablation with a carbon dioxide laser.

Condyloma Acuminatum (Venereal Wart) (Figs. 37-5 and 37-6) The condyloma acuminatum is a transmissible papillomatous growth that may look identical to the papilloma or fibroma, except for several distinguishing features. The oral condyloma occurs much less frequently than the papilloma. It is seen more commonly in sexually active individuals and is much more likely to be multiple. The warm, moist, intertriginous areas of the anogenital skin and mucosa are frequent sites of growth.

Condyloma acuminata are usually multiple, small, and colored pink to dirty gray. The surface may be flat, but is more often pebbly and resembles a cauliflower. The base is sessile and the borders are raised and rounded. Contagious spread may occur among the host and sexual partners. When multiple lesions are present, proliferation of adjacent condylomas can form extensive clusters that may appear as a single mass. Any oral mucosal surface may be affected, but the labial mucosa is the most common site. Histologically condylomata exhibit parakeratosis, cryptic invagination of cornified cells, and koilocytosis. Over 85% of condyloma acuminata have HPV Types 6 and 11 DNA present in the epithelium. Treatment of choice is wide excision, since these lesions have a high rate of recurrence. Occasional oncogenic transformation of long-standing growths has been reported.

Lymphangioma (Figs. 37-7 and 37-8) Lymphangiomas are benign tumors of lymphatic channels that develop early in life with no sexual predilection. They may occur on skin or mucous membrane. The oral cavity is a frequent site. The most common intraoral site is the dorsal and lateral surface of the anterior portion of the tongue, followed by the lips and labial mucosa.

Small superficial lymphangiomas have irregular papillary projections that resemble a papilloma. They are soft and compressible, and vary in color from normal pink to whitish, slightly translucent, or blue. Deep-seated lesions cause diffuse enlargement and stretching of the surface mucosa. Macroglossia, macrocheilia, and cystic hygroma are clinical deformities resulting from the diffuse swelling.

Aspiration or diascopy is mandatory prior to surgical excision of a lymphangioma to prevent complications associated with the similar-appearing hemangioma. Patients with a large, diffuse lesion often require hopitalization to monitor post-operative edema and possible airway obstruction. Lymphangiomas do not undergo malignant change. Some lymphangiomas, especially congenital types, regress spontaneously during childhood.

PAPULONODULES

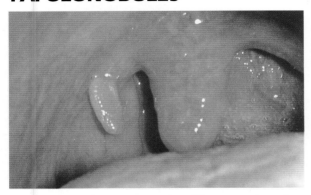

Fig. 37-1. Pedunculated pink **papilloma** on the soft palate. (Courtesy Dr Curt Lundeen)

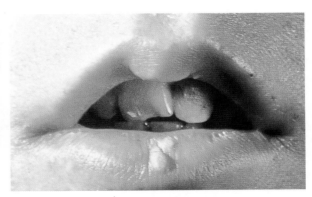

Fig. 37-2. Firm whitish **verruca vulgaris.**

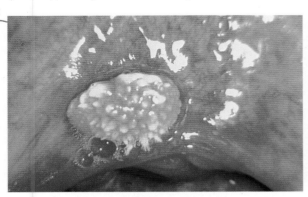

Fig. 37-3. Whitish **papilloma** with surface projections on the soft palate. (Courtesy Dr Tom McDavid)

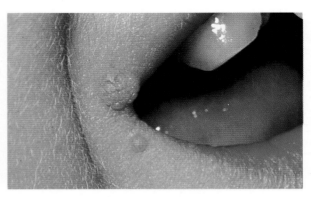

Fig. 37-4. Multiple **verrucae vulgaris** at commissure of the lips.

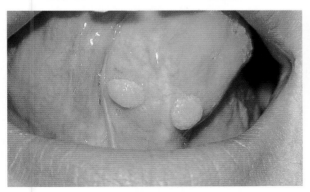

Fig. 37-5. Papular **condyloma acuminata** on ventral tongue.

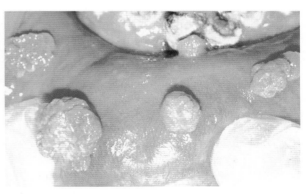

Fig. 37-6. Multiple grayish-pink **condyloma acuminata.**

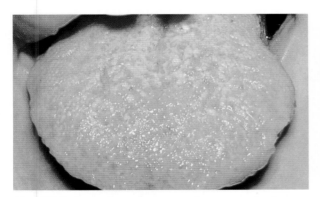

Fig. 37-7. Lymphangioma causing macroglossia.

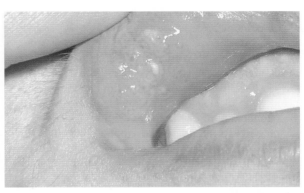

Fig. 37-8. Papulonodular surface of a **lymphagioma** of the lip in the same patient as in Fig. 37-7.

VESICULOBULLOUS LESIONS

Primary Herpetic Gingivostomatitis (Figs. 38-1 through 38-3) Herpes simplex virus (HSV) Types 1 and 2 belong to the family Herpesviridae, which also includes cytomegalovirus, varicella zoster virus, and Epstein-Barr and the recently discovered human herpes virus VI. These viruses are ubiquitous in nature and infect a wide variety of animal species.

Approximately 80 to 90% of the adult human population have been infected with HSV. Viral transmission occurs by direct mucocutaneous contact of infected secretions, resulting in over half of a million cases of primary herpetic gingivostomatitis annually in the United States. HSV-1 is the causative organism in the majority of cases; however, Type 2 herpes virus, which has a propensity to infect the skin below the waist, can cause herpetic gingivostomatitis by oral-genital or oral-oral contact.

The manifestations of the primary infection may be trivial or fulminating. Trivial infections may produce subclinical signs of infection that often go unrecognized, or flu-like symptoms. The initial infection of herpetic gingivostomatitis primarily affects children under the age of 10, and secondarily young adults aged 15 to 25 years.

The acute inflammatory response of the primary infection of HSV usually follows a 3- to 10-day incubation period. The infected individual will complain of fever, malaise, and irritability. Initially, focal areas of the marginal gingiva become fiery red and edematous. The swollen interdental papillae bleed after minute trauma because of capillary fragility and increased permeability. Widespread inflammation of the marginal and attached gingiva develops, and small clusters of vesicles rapidly erupt throughout the mouth. The vesicles burst, forming yellowish ulcers that are individually circumscribed by a red-halo. Coalescence of adjacent lesions forms large ulcers of the buccal mucosa, labial mucosa, gingiva, palate, tongue, and lips. Shallow erosions of the perioral skin may be apparent. Hemorrhagic crusts of the lips are characteristic. Headache, lymphadenopathy, and pharyngitis are usually present.

A significant problem in patients with primary herpetic gingivostomatitis is the pain caused by the mouth ulcers. Mastication and deglutition may be impared, resulting in dehydration and subsequent elevation of temperature. Viral culturing, serum antibodies, and cytology are confirmatory. Treatment is supportive and should include acyclovir in severe cases.

Primary herpetic gingivostomatitis is a contagious disease that usually regresses spontaneously within 12 to 20 days without scarring. Complications associated with the primary infection include auto-inoculation of other epidermal sites, producing keratoconjunctivitis and herpetic whitlow; extensive epidermal infection in the atopic individual, which is termed Kaposi's varicelliform eruption; meningitis, encephalitis, and disseminated infections in immunosuppressed patients. Immunity to HSV is relative, and patients previously infected with the virus may be reinfected with a different strain of HSV.

Recurrent Herpes Simplex (Figs. 38-4 through 38-7) Following the initial infection, HSV infects sensory nerve fibers, migrates to a regional neuronal ganglia, and becomes stably associated with the nucleus of the infected cell in a latent and undetectable manner. Reactivation of virus, replication of progeny particles, and clinical recurrence occurs in approximately 40% of persons that harbor the latent virus. Recrudescence is dependent on the ability of immune mechanisms to eliminate reactivated HSV. Recurrences are often precipitated by a triggering event such as sunlight, heat, stress, trauma, or immunosuppression.

Recurrent herpes simplex (RHS) tends to produce clusters of vesicles that ulcerate. The vesicles repeatedly develop at the same site following the distribution of the infected nerve. Recurrences on the vermilion border of the lip (recurrent herpes labialis) are clinically more apparent than intraoral recurrences (recurrent herpetic stomatitis).The lesions of recurrent herpes labialis are characterized by the appearance of small clusters of vesicles that erupt, coalesce, and form slightly depressed, yellow-brown ulcers that have distinct red halos. Spread to perioral skin is common, especially if greasy lip ointments are used that permit horizontal weeping of vesicular fluid. Contact of infected fluid with other epidermal structures can result in autoinoculation of the eye (keratoconjunctivitis), finger (herpetic whitlow), or genitalia (genital herpes). In relatively healthy persons, recurrent herpetic stomatitis is limited to periosteal-bound, keratinized mucosa consisting of the attached gingiva and hard palate. Recurrences on the buccal mucosa and tongue are infrequent, unless the patient is immunosuppressed.

Most patients with RHS complain of pain, although some individuals experience little discomfort. Prodromal neurogenic symptoms such as tingling, throbbing, and burning often precede the eruption of lesions by 24 hours. Sunscreens are effective in the prevention of recurrences. Management also includes lysine, vitamin C, and antiviral drugs (acyclovir) in the immunosuppressed.

Herpangina (Fig. 38-8) Herpangina is a self limiting infection involving the oral cavity, caused by group A Coxsackie viruses. This infection is seen mainly in children during the warmer months of summer, and is highly contagious. Young adults are occasionally affected. Herpangina produces light-gray papillary vesicles that rupture to form multiple, discrete, shallow ulcers. The ulcers have an erythematous border and are limited to the anterior pillars of the fauces, soft palate, uvula, and the tonsils. Diffuse pharyngeal erythema, dysphagia, and sore throat are common features, as are fever, malaise, headache, lymphadenitis, abdominal pain, and vomiting. Convulsions rarely occur. Treatment is palliative and spontaneous healing occurs within 1 to 2 weeks.

VESICULOBULLOUS LESIONS

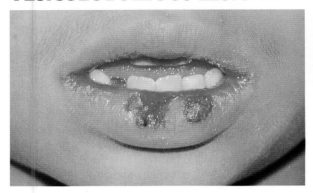

Fig. 38-1. Crusting lips; **primary herpetic gingivo-stomatitis.**

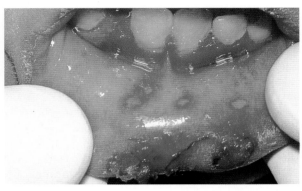

Fig. 38-2. Multiple broken-down **herpetic vesicles** with red halos; same patient as in Fig. 38-1.

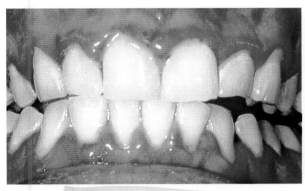

Fig. 38-3. **Primary infection of herpes simplex virus type I** producing painful gingivitis.

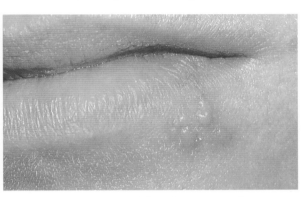

Fig. 38-4. Virus-laden vesicles of **recurrent herpes labialis.** (Courtesy Dr James Cottone)

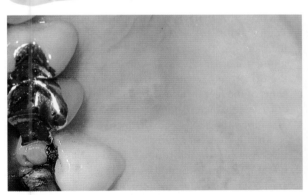

Fig. 38-5. **Recurrent herpes simplex** of the palate.

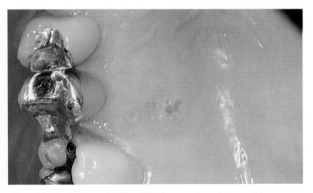

Fig. 38-6. Patient in Fig. 38-5 two days later with broken down **herpetic vesicles.**

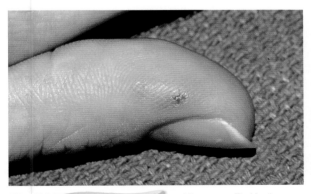

Fig. 38-7. **Herpetic whitlow.** (Courtesy Dr Linda Otis)

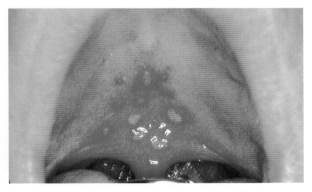

Fig. 38-8. Erythematous soft palate with multiple vesicles; **herpangina.** (Courtesy Dr Charles Morris)

85

VESICULOBULLOUS LESIONS

Varicella (Chickenpox) (Figs. 39-1 and 39-2)
Varicella and herpes zoster are caused by the same herpetic virus, varicella zoster. Varicella is the highly contagious primary infection, whereas herpes zoster is the recurrent neurodermal infection. Typically, young children become infected with the, virus during the late winter and spring months. Following exposure to the virus and a 2 to 3 week incubation period, mild prodromal features appear.

Fever, malaise, and a distinctive red rash on the trunk are the first recognizable signs of this disease. The pruritic rash quickly spreads to the neck, face and extremities, and is followed shortly by the eruption of papules that form vesicles and pustules. Individual vesicles burst, producing a "dew drop on a rose petal" appearance. The first and largest skin lesion is called the "herald spot." It is often located on the face and, if scratched, may heal with scarring.

Intraoral lesions of varicella are few and often go unnoticed. They appear as vesicular lesions that break down and form ulcers with an erythematous halo. The soft palate is the predominant site, followed by the buccal mucosa and mucobuccal fold. Anorexia, chills, fever, nasopharyngitis, and musculoskeletal aches may accompany the course of the disease. Complications are infrequent, and vesicles eventually crust over and resolve spontaneously within 7 to 10 days. Infection during pregnancy poses a significant risk to the fetus.

Herpes Zoster (Shingles) (Figs. 39-3 and 39-4)
Herpes zoster is the recurrent infection of chickenpox. Unknown factors result in reactivation of dormant varicella virus from sensory ganglia and migration of virus along the affected sensory nerves. Viral recrudescence usually affects older adults past age 50, but may be seen in young adults or children. Prior to eruption, prodromal signs of itching, tingling, burning, pain, or paresthesia occur. Lesions are characterized by acutely painful vesicular eruptions of the skin and mucosa that are unilaterally distributed along nerve pathways and stop abruptly at the midline. Two areas are affected the most: the trunk between vertebras T3 and L2, and the face along the ophthalmic division of the trigeminal nerve.

Cutaneous lesions of shingles begin as erythematous macules that are followed by vesicular and pustular eruptions. Crust formation occurs within 7 to 10 days and persists for several weeks. Pain is intense, but usually dissipates when the crusts fall off.

The intraoral lesions are vesicular and ulcerative with an intense red, inflammatory border. A hemorrhagic component is common. The lips, tongue, and buccal mucosa may have unilateral ulcerative lesions if the mandibular branch of the trigeminal nerve is affected. Involvement of the second division of the trigeminal nerve typically produces unilateral palatal ulcerations that extend up to but not beyond the palatal raphe. Considerable malaise, fever, and distress accompany herpes zoster. Patients often present with intense pain 1 to 2 days before the viral vesicles erupt.

Herpes zoster usually heals without scar formation within about 3 weeks, but many patients may experience persistent pain after the lesions have faded. This condition, called "postherpetic neuralgia," may continue for 6 months to a year before regressing. It is resistant to most forms of therapy. Patients who are immunosuppressed are particularly susceptible to shingles and have a high morbidity rate. In the past the rare occurrence of bilateral shingles was termed "the death sign" because these victims inevitably died. Varicella zoster virus infection is occasionally associated with the Ramsay Hunt syndrome (herpes zoster, unilateral facial paralysis, and ear eruptions) and Reye's syndrome (high fever, cerebral edema, liver degeneration, high mortality, and salicylate use).

Hand-Foot-and-Mouth Disease (Figs. 39-5 through 39-8)
Hand-foot-and-mouth disease is a mildly contagious disease caused by a number of Coxsackie A and B viruses. It usually affects children, but may be seen in young adults. It typically occurs in spring and summer. As the name implies, it produces small ulcerative lesions in the mouth together with an erythematous and vascular rash on the dorsal and ventral surface of the hands, fingers, and soles of the feet. Multiple pinpoint vesicles that ulcerate and crust are characteristic. There may be several to more than 100 pinpoint lesions with distinctive erythematous halos.

Oral lesions of hand-foot-and-mouth disease are scattered mainly on the tongue, hard palate, and buccal and labial mucosa. In time they coalesce to form large eroded areas. The oropharynx is usually unaffected. The total number of intraoral lesions is usually less than 20. Pain is a common symptom, along with elevated temperature, malaise, and lymphadenopathy. The diagnosis can be made by viral culture and serum antibody studies; however, the classic distribution of lesions on the palms of hands, soles of feet, and oral mucosa is diagnostic in most instances. Healing occurs regardless of treatment in approximately 10 days.

VESICULOBULLOUS LESIONS

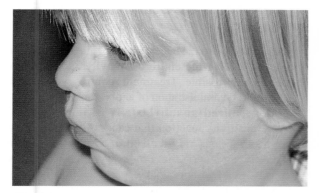

Fig. 39-1. Maculopapular facial rash of **chickenpox.**

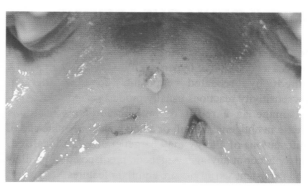

Fig. 39-2. Intraoral vesicle of **chickenpox.**

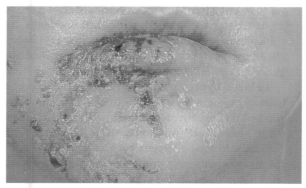

Fig. 39-3. Unilateral eruption of **herpes zoster** along the mandibular branch of the trigeminal nerve.

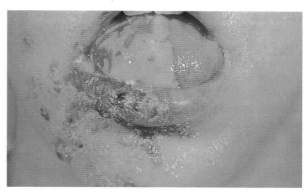

Fig. 39-4. Painful intraoral lesions of patient in Fig. 39-3 with **herpes zoster.**

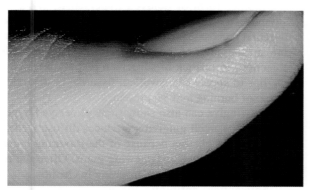

Fig. 39-5. Typical pinpoint lesion of **hand-foot-and-mouth disease** in a young adult. (Courtesy Drs Birgit & Tom Glass)

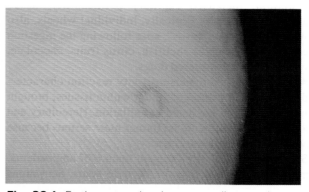

Fig. 39-6. Erythematous border surrounding an ulcer; **hand-foot-and-mouth disease.** (Courtesy Drs Birgit & Tom Glass)

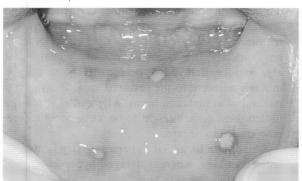

Fig. 39-7. Hand-foot-and-mouth disease of the labial mucosa. (Courtesy Drs Birgit & Tom Glass)

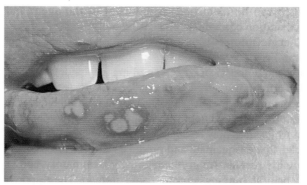

Fig. 39-8. Painful clusters of vesicles of **hand-foot-and-mouth disease;** same patient in Figs. 39-5 through 39-8. (Courtesy Drs Birgit & Tom Glass)

VESICULOBULLOUS LESIONS

Erythema Multiforme (Figs. 41-1 through 41-4)

Erythema multiforme is a self-limiting disease of the skin and mucous membranes. It commonly affects young adults, particularly males, but may affect children and the elderly as well. Low-grade fever, malaise, and headache typically precede the emergence of lesions by 3 to 7 days.

Erythema multiforme has an unknown etiology; however, recent evidence suggest that circulating immune complexes that provoke complement-mediated cytopathic effects, combined with lymphocytic and neutrophilic stimulated vascular injury, may play a pathogenic role. Precipitating factors include bacterial, fungal, and viral infections such as herpes simplex and *Mycoplasma pneumoniae,* emotional stress, and allergy, especially to sulfa- and barbiturate-containing drugs. In about 50% of the cases no causative factor has been identified.

Although there is great variation in the clinical appearance of the disease, as the name "multiforme" suggests, stomatitis and cutaneous lesions are the most prominent features. The hallmarks of this disease are the red-white, concentric, ring-like macules termed "target," "bulls-eye," or "iris" lesions that rapidly appear on the extensor surfaces of the arms and legs, knees, and palms of the hands. The trunk of the body is classically exempt from lesions, except in the most severe cases.

Initially the skin lesions are small, red, circular macules that vary in size from 0.5 to 2.0 cm in diameter. Then the macules enlarge and develop a pale white or central clear area. Shortly thereafter the lesions form vesicles and bullae. The vesicles may go unnoticed until they rupture and become confluent. The ulcers formed are large, raw, and shallow, with an erythematous border. A necrotic slough and a fibrinous pseudomembrane typically cover the ulcers. Urticarial plaques that do not break down may also be present.

Intraorally, red macular areas, multiple ulcerations, and erosions with a gray-white fibrinous surface may be seen. They are limited to the buccal mucosa, labial mucosa, palate, or tongue, or involve all of those areas. Rarely is the gingiva involved. Dark, red-brown, hemorrhagic crusts are characteristically present on the lips, which aids in making the diagnosis. Lesions are usually short-lived and last about 2 weeks. Erythema multiforme rarely persists for more than 1 month. Oral lesions without cutaneous lesions have been reported. Recurrent and chronic forms exist.

Pain is the most common symptom, which may interfere with normal oral activity. Oral hygiene may be neglected, resulting in secondary bacterial infection. Treatment consists of topical palliative rinses and, in some instances, low dose systemic steroids. Complications resulting from erythema multiforme are uncommon unless the disease progresses to its major form, Stevens-Johnson syndrome.

Stevens-Johnson Syndrome (Figs. 41-5 through 41-8)

The severe form or major variant of erythema multiforme is termed "Stevens-Johnson syndrome," named for the two investigators who first described the clinical appearance of the disease in the early 1920s. It frequently affects children and young adults, predominantly males. The oral signs of Stevens-Johnson syndrome are similar to those of erythema multiforme, but there is more widespread involvement of cutaneous and stomatologic structures, together with more constitutional signs including fever, malaise, headache, cough, chest pain, diarrhea, vomiting, and arthralgia.

The classic clinical triad of Stevens-Johnson syndrome consists of eye lesions (conjunctivitis), genital lesions (balanitis, vulvovaginitis), and stomatitis. In addition there are the characteristic target skin lesions on the face, chest, and abdomen that later develop into painful "weeping" vesiculobullous lesions.

Like erythema multiforme, the gingiva is less commonly affected by desquamating bullae than the non-keratinized mucosa. Extensive ulcerative and hemorrhagic lesions of the lips and denuded areas of oral mucosa are intensely painful and usually prevent affected patients from eating and swallowing. Inadequate nutritional intake, dehydration, and debilitation are common sequelae that necessitate hospitalization.

Significant morbidity and mortality may occur if supportive therapy is not provided. Treatment consists of intravenous fluid and nutritional therapy, short-term corticosteroids, and palliation consisting of oral anesthetic rinses, agents that coat and protect the lesions, and antiseptic mouthwashes. Secondary infection is managed with antibiotics, the ensuing fever with fluids and antipyretics. The condition has a longer duration than erythema multiforme, but usually resolves within 6 weeks. Fatalities have been documented in sulfa-induced Stevens-Johnson syndrome.

VESICULOBULLOUS LESIONS

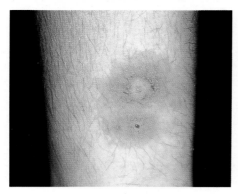

Fig. 41-1. Target lesion; **erythema multiforme.** (Courtesy Dr Tom McDavid)

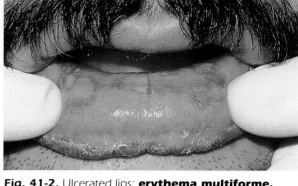

Fig. 41-2. Ulcerated lips; **erythema multiforme.** (Courtesy Dr John McDowell)

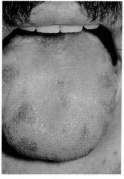

Fig. 41-3. Multiple erythematous ulcers on the dorsum of the tongue; **erythema multiforme.** (Courtesy Dr John McDowell)

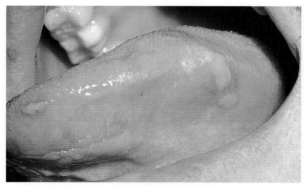

Fig. 41-4. Ulcers of **erythema multiforme** on ventral tongue; same patient in Figs. 41-2 through 41-4. (Courtesy Dr John McDowell)

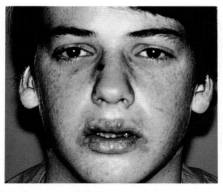

Fig. 41-5. Stevens-Johnson syndrome. (Courtesy Dr Tom McDavid)

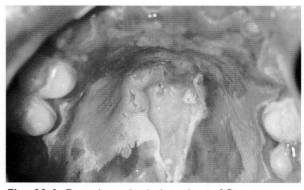

Fig. 41-6. Extensive palatal ulcerations of **Stevens-Johnson syndrome** in same patient as in Fig. 41-5. (Courtesy Dr Tom McDavid)

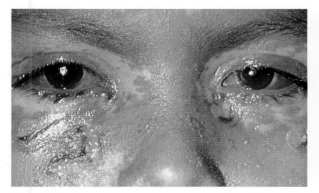

Fig. 41-7. Severe conjunctivitis and weeping skin lesions; **Stevens-Johnson syndrome.**

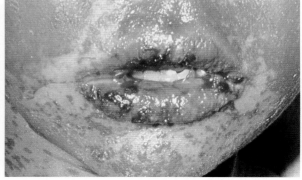

Fig. 41-8. Hemorragic and crusted lips of child seen in Fig. 41-7 who has **Stevens-Johnson syndrome.**

VESICULOBULLOUS LESIONS

Pemphigus Vulgaris (Figs. 42-1 through 42-4)

Pemphigus is a potentially fatal, vesiculobullous disease which has been categorized into four types: **vulgaris** and **vegetans,** which have intraoral manifestations, and **foliaceous** and **erythematosus,** which are not believed to produce oral disease. The most important aspect of this condition is early recognition of the oral lesions, which usually precede skin involvement by several months. In fact, oral lesions may be the only manifestation of the disease. Diagnosis during the early stages greatly enhances the initiation of corticosteroid and immunosuppressive therapy and, therefore, the long-term prognosis.

Vulgaris, the most common type of intraoral pemphigus, usually develops between the ages of 30 and 50. It may be seen in younger or older patients, but rarely does it develop in patients beyond 60 years. It is seen with equal frequency in males and females and is usually encountered in light-pigmented patients of Jewish or Mediterranean origin. Pemphigus vulgaris is probably an autoimmune disorder involving a reaction of IgG to an intercellular subtance, resulting in epithelial cell-to-cell separation. Acute and chronic forms exist, the slow chronic form being the most common.

The most prominent clinical feature of pemphigus is the rapid development of multiple bullae that tend to rupture and leave erosions of the skin and oral mucous membranes. When there is systemic involvement, severe debilitation may result in death. Early mucocutaneous lesions consist of "weeping" bullae or gelatinous plaques that are clear and shimmering. The bullae are extremely fragile and rapidly disintegrate, hemorrhage, and crust. They tend to recur in the same area and later spread to adjacent regions. Light lateral pressure applied to a bulla will cause it to enlarge by extension (Nikolsky's sign). A characteristic and consistent finding is the appearance of a whitish superficial covering, which is the roof of a collapsed bulla that can easily be stripped away. Cases that show predominantly desquamative areas that affect the gingiva have been clinically termed "desquamative gingivitis."

Pemphigus may appear as an epithelial slough with white tissue folds, an aphthous or traumatic ulcer or, in circumstances involving multiple areas of the lips, buccal mucosa, tongue, gingiva, palate, and oropharynx, the condition may resemble erythema multiforme. Individual lesions often have circular or serpiginous borders, whereas extensive erosions of the buccal mucosa are red and raw, and have diffuse irregular borders. Frequent eruptions may be superimposed over healing lesions so that periods of remission are absent. The tongue is less commonly involved than the lips, buccal mucosa, and gingiva. Thick hemorrhagic crusts and fetor oris are characteristic of extensive lesions. Patients with pemphigus are often disturbed by the severe pain associated with the condition.

The diagnosis of pemphigus is confirmed by a positive Nikolsky's sign, biopsy, and immunofluorescent staining techniques. Prior to steroid therapy, dehydration and septicemia were fatal complications of pemphigus.

Benign Mucous Membrane (Cicatricial) Pemphigoid and Bullous Pemphigoid (Figs. 42-5 through 42-8)

Pemphigoid is a chronic, self-limiting, mucocutaneous disease that is slightly more common in the oral cavity than pemphigus, but is associated with much less morbidity and mortality. Two types that produce identical oral lesions may be seen in the mouth: benign mucous membrane pemphigoid and bullous pemphigoid.

Bullous pemphigoid, which is the least common of the two, affects both the skin and the oral cavity, and has no sexual or racial predisposition. Skin folds located at the axilla, inguinal, and abdominal regions are commonly affected. The second type, benign mucous membrane pemphigoid (BMMP), also termed "cicatricial," is limited to the mucous membranes, favoring the ocular and oral membranes. This disease occurs twice as frequently in women than men usually after the age of 50. Occasionally younger persons are affected. There is no racial predilection.

Pemphigoid skin lesions usually precede oral lesions, tend to be desquamative and localized, and heal spontaneously. The lips are rarely affected. Intraoral bullae are usually small tense blebs that are yellow or hemorrhagic. They form slowly and tend to favor the palate, gingiva, and buccal mucosa. Because bullae of pemphigoid result from a subepithelial separation, they are thicker-walled, less fragile, and longer-lasting than those of pemphigus. In some instances patients may have bullae that persist for several days before rupture, and it is this intactness that suggests the diagnosis of pemphigoid. Large, shallow ulcers can result from coalescence of several adjacent lesions. The ulcers are surrounded by an erythematous ring, exhibit a symmetrical pattern, and occasionally bleed.

When the condition is limited to the gingiva, which occurs frequently, the clinical term "desquamative gingivitis" has been used to describe the bright, red, burning and denuded gingiva. "Desquamative gingivitis" is a descriptive term and may represent several clinically similar conditions such as erosive lichen planus, pemphigoid, and pemphigus for which a diagnosis is not yet obtained.

BMMP may affect the anal, vaginal, and pharyngeal mucosa, but the most severe complication of BMMP is ocular involvement producing conjunctivitis, occasional bullae, clouding of the cornea, and fibrous scarring. Blindness is a serious sequela of protracted eye disease.

Although pemphigoid is rarely fatal, close followup is suggested for progressive cases, since carcinoma of the rectum and uterus have been associated with this disorder. Moderate doses of corticosteroids alone, or in conjunction with immunosuppressive agents such as azathioprine, have provided effective management.

VESICULOBULLOUS LESIONS

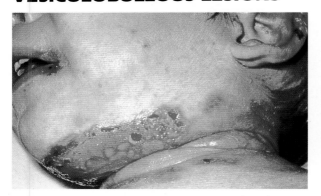

Fig. 42-1. Young child with extensive erosions of **pemphigus vulgaris.**

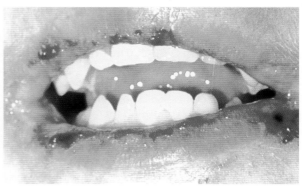

Fig. 42-2. Lip involvement of child in Fig. 42-1 with **pemphigus vulgaris.**

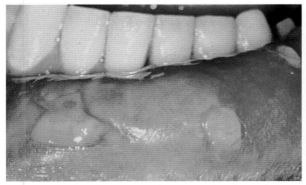

Fig. 42-3. Superficial clear bullae of **pemphigus vulgaris.** (Courtesy Drs Tom McDavid and Martin Tyler)

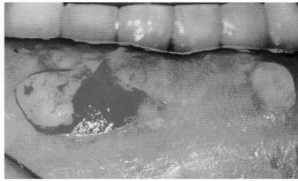

Fig. 42-4. Ruptured and hemorrhagic bullae; **pemphigus vulgaris.** (Courtesy Drs Tom McDavid and Martin Tyler)

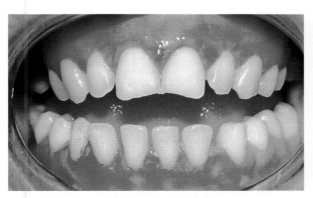

Fig. 42-5. "Desquamative gingivitis"; **benign mucous membrane pemphigoid.**

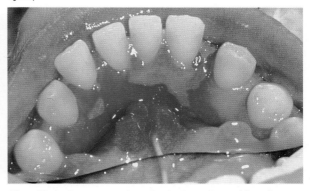

Fig. 42-6. Desquamative gingival patches of **benign mucous membrane pemphigoid.**

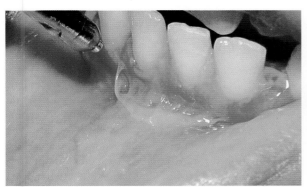

Fig. 42-7. Nikolsky's sign suggestive of **benign mucous membrane pemphigoid;** same patient in Figs. 42-5 through 42-7.

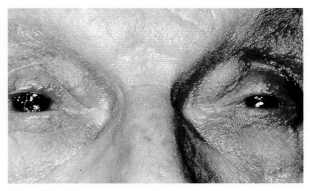

Fig. 42-8. Corneal scarring; **benign mucous membrane pemphigoid.**

ULCERATIVE LESIONS

Traumatic Ulcer (Figs. 43-1 through 43-3) Recurrent oral ulceration is a common condition resulting from several etiologies, trauma being the most common cause. Ulcers may occur at any age and in either sex. Likely locations for traumatic ulcers are the labial mucosa, buccal mucosa, palate, and peripheral borders of the tongue.

Traumatic ulcers may result from chemicals, heat, electricity, or mechanical force, and are often classified according to the exact nature of the insult. Pressure from an ill-fitting denture base or flange, or from a partial denture framework, is a source of a decubitous or pressure ulcer. Trophic, or ischemic ulcers, occur particularly on the palate at the site of a previous injection. Dental injections have also been implicated in the traumatic ulcerations seen on the lower lip by children who chew their lip after dental appointments. In addition to factitial injury, young children and infants are prone to traumatic ulcers of the soft palate from thumb sucking, called Bednar's aphthae.

Ulcers may be precipitated by contact with a fractured tooth, a partial denture clasp, or inadvertent biting of the mucosa. A burn from food or drinks that are too hot commonly occurs on the palate. Other traumatic ulcers are caused by factitial injury from inappropriate use of fingernails on the oral mucosa. The diagnosis of these conditions is simple and is often obtained from a careful history and examination of the physical findings.

The appearance of a mechanically induced traumatic ulcer varies according to the intensity and size of the agent. The ulcer usually appears slightly depressed and oval in shape. Initially an erythematous zone is found at the periphery, which progressively lightens because of the keratinization process. The center of the ulcer is usually yellow-gray. Chemically damaged mucosa, such as that with an aspirin burn, is less well-defined and contains a loosely adherent, coagulated surface slough. Following removal of the traumatic influence, the ulcer should heal within 2 weeks, if not other causes should be suspected and a biopsy performed.

Recurrent Aphthous Stomatitis (Minor Aphthae, Aphthous Ulcer) (Figs. 43-4 through 43-6)

Recurrent aphthous stomatitis (RAS) is classified into three categories according to size: minor aphthae, major aphthae, and herpetiform ulcers. Approximately 20% of the population is afflicted with minor aphthae, or "canker sores" as they are commonly referred to by patients. They may be seen in anyone, but females and young adults are slightly more susceptible. Familial patterns have been demonstrated and persons who smoke are less frequently affected than non-smokers. Factors that precipitate aphthae include atopy, trauma, endocrinopathies, menstruation, nutritional deficiences, stress, and food allergies. Although the etiology is unknown, current studies suggest an immunopathic process involving cell-mediated cytolytic activity in response to HLA or foreign antigens. The L-form of streptococcus has been suggested to play a causal role in the formation of aphthous ulceration.

Minor aphthous ulcers have a propensity for movable mucosa that is situated over minor salivary gland tissue. The labial and buccal mucosa are frequently affected, whereas ulcers are rarely seen on heavily keratinized mucosa such as the gingiva and hard palate. Occasionally, prodromal symptoms of paresthesia or hyperesthesia are reported.

Minor aphthae appear as shallow, yellow-gray, oval ulcers usually about 2 to 5 mm in diameter. A prominent erythematous border surrounds the fibrinous pseudomembrane. No vesicle formation is seen in this disease, a distinctive diagnostic feature. Ulcers that occur along the mucobuccal fold often appear more elongated.

Burning is a preliminary complaint that is followed by intense pain of a few days' duration. Tender submandibular, anterior cervical, and parotid nodes are often present, particularly when the ulcer becomes secondarily infected.

Aphthae are invariably, recurrent, and the pattern of occurrence varies. Most persons exhibit single ulcers, once or twice a year, beginning during childhood or adolescence. Occasionally the ulcers appear in crops, but usually less than five occur at one time. Patients with multiple ulcers may have periods of several months in which the ulcers are constant. Persistent ulcerations are often extremely painful and usually have a ragged appearance. More extreme measures may be required to effectively treat those patients. Minor aphthous ulcers usually heal spontaneously without scar formation within 14 days.

Although no medication has been totally successful in the treatment of aphthous stomatitis, patients have responded to antibiotic suspensions and coagulating, cauterizing, and anti-inflammatory agents.

Pseudoaphthous Ulcer (Figs. 43-7 and 43-8)

Pseudoaphthae is a term coined by Binney that refers to recurrent, aphthous-like mucosal ulcers of the mouth, which are associated with nutritional deficiency states. Studies indicate that 20% of patients with recurrent aphthous stomatitis are deficient in folic acid, iron, or vitamin B_{12}. Pseudoaphthae are frequently concomitant with inflammatory bowel disease, Crohn's disease, gluten intolerance, and pernicious anemia.

Pseudoaphthae resemble aphthous ulcers, but are characteristically more persistent. There is a slight predilection for females between the ages of 25 and 50. The ulcers are depressed, rounded, and painful. The borders may be raised and firm, but induration is seldom encountered. Alterations of the tongue papillae may clue the diagnostician of an underlying nutritional deficiency state. Healing is slow, and patients may complain of never being free of ulceration. Chronic and persistent disease necessitates evaluation for nutritional deficiencies, including hematologic studies. If the laboratory results are abnormal then a medical referral is required.

ULCERATIVE LESIONS

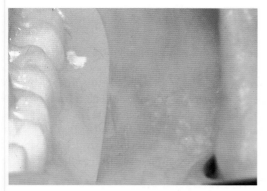

Fig. 43-1. Denture-flange-induced **traumatic ulcer.**

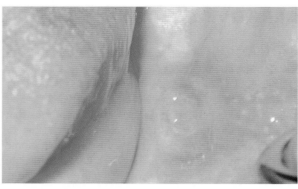

Fig. 43-2. Traumatic ulcer; *same patient as in Fig. 43-1.*

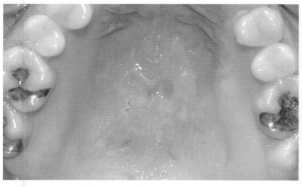

Fig. 43-3. Traumatic ulcer due to the ingestion of burning-hot food. (Courtesy Dr Donna Wood)

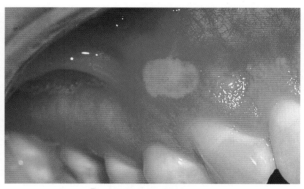

Fig. 43-4. Oval **aphthous ulcer** on alveolar mucosa.

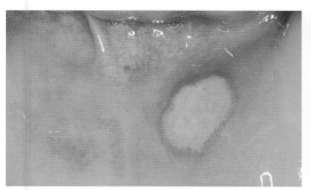

Fig. 43-5. Aphthous ulcer with prominent red border on labial mucosa. (Courtesy Dr Tom Schiff)

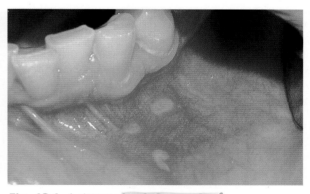

Fig. 43-6. A cluster of **aphthous ulcers.**

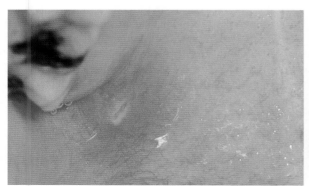

Fig. 43-7. A wide band of erythema surrounding a palatal ulcer in a patient with **Crohn's disease.** (Courtesy Dr Donna Wood)

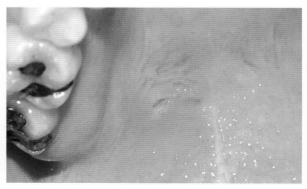

Fig. 43-8. Pseudoaphthous ulcer of Crohn's disease. (Courtesy Dr Donna Wood)

ULCERATIVE LESIONS

Major Aphthous (Peridadenitis Mucosa Necrotica Recurrens [PMNR], Sutton's Disease, Scarifying Stomatitis, Recurrent Scarring Aphthous Ulcer) (Figs. 44-1 through 44-4) Major aphthous is an exaggerated variant of minor aphthous that produces larger and more destructive ulcers that last longer and recur more frequently. The etiology is unknown; some suggest that an immune defect is involved. Others speculate that the large ulcer is a severe form of recurrent aphthous stomatitis, which results from the coalescence of several smaller ulcers. Young female adults with anxious personality traits are most commonly affected.

Major aphthous ulcerations are often multiple. They involve the soft palate, tonsillar fauces, labial mucosa, buccal mucosa, and tongue, occasionally extending onto the attached gingiva. Characteristically the ulcers are asymmetric and unilateral. The most prominent feature is the large size together with a depressed, necrotic center. A red raised inflammatory border is common. Depending on size, traumatic influences, and secondary infection, ulcers may last from several weeks to months. Because the ulcers erode deep into the connective tissue, they heal with scar formation and tissue distortion. Muscle destruction can result in tissue fenestration, and if the periodontium is involved, loss of tissue attachment may occur. Extreme pain and lymphadenopathy are common symptoms.

Healing can be accelerated and scarring reduced with the use of steroids. Ulcers similar to those of PMNR are seen with some frequency in association with cyclic neutropenia, agranulocytosis, and gluten intolerance. Ulcers located on the tongue may strongly resemble carcinoma. The presence of scarring is of diagnostic importance to rule out malignancy.

Herpetiform Ulceration (Figs. 44-5 and 44-6) Herpetiform ulceration is a type of recurrent focal ulceration of the oral mucosa that clinically resembles the ulcers seen in primary herpes; hence the name herpetiform. This condition, however, is probably a variant form of recurrent aphthous ulceration. The prominent feature of the disease is the numerous, pinhead-sized, gray-white erosions that enlarge, coalesce, and become ill-defined. Initially the ulcers are 1 to 2 mm in diameter and occur in clusters of 10 to 100. The mucosa adjacent to the ulcer is erythematous, and pain is a predictable symptom.

Any part of the oral mucosa may be affected by herpetiform ulcerations, but particularly affected is the anterior tip of the tongue, margins of the tongue, and labial mucosa. The smaller size of these ulcerations distinguishes them from aphthae, while their absence of vesicles and gingivitis together with their recurrent nature distinguishes them from primary herpes and other oral viral infections. Virus cannot be cultured from these lesions, and the ulcers are not contagious.

The first episode of herpetiform ulceration usually occurs in patients in their late twenties, 10 years after the peak incidence of aphthae. The duration of the attack is variable and unpredictable, and the etiology has yet to be determined. Recurrent herpetiform ulcerations respond especially well to tetracycline suspensions, and the condition often regresses spontaneously after several years.

Behçet's Syndrome (Oculo-Oral-Genital Syndrome) (Figs. 44-7 and 44-8) Behçet's syndrome, named for the Turkish physician who first described the ulcerative disorder, principally involves three sites: the eye, oral cavity, and genitals. For this reason it has been categorized as a triple-symptom complex with ulcerative manifestations. In its fully developed state, cutaneous lesions, arthritis of the major joints, gastrointestinal ulcerations, neurologic manifestations, and thrombophlebitis can be seen, though rarely are all components present in the same patient. The etiology remains unknown, but a delayed hypersensitivity reaction, possibly involving HLA antigens, immune complexes, and vasculitis, has been suggested.

Behçet's syndrome is two to three times more prevalent in males than in females, with an onset between the ages of 20 and 30. Persons from Asia, the Mediterranean coast, and Great Britain are most commonly affected.

Eye manifestations of Behçet's syndrome include photophobia, conjunctivitis, and chronic recurrent iritis with hypopyon that occasionally leads to blindness. Ocular manifestations may be concurrent with or occur years after oral and genital ulcers. Skin changes are characterized by subcutaneous nodules and macular and papular eruptions that vesiculate, ulcerate, and encrustate. Genital ulcers may involve the mucosa or skin, and tend to be smaller and less common than the oral lesions.

Oral ulcers, the most prevalent lesion of Behçet's syndrome, may be the initial sign of the disease. One, a few, or crops of aphthous-like ulcers on the buccal or labial mucosa are characteristic; however, any oral mucosal site may be involved. Similar to aphthous, the ulcers are flat, shallow, and oval, with the size of the ulcers varying. Small lesions tend to occur more frequently than larger lesions. A serofibrinous exudate covers the surface, and the margins are red and well-demarcated. Complaints of pain are frequent, and recurrent periods of exacerbation and remissions are characteristic. Patients with limited mucocutaneous involvement are managed symptomatically with topical and systemic steroids. Protracted disease involving the neuro-ocular structures requires the care of a physician. Azathioprine, cyclophosphamide, thalidomide, and colchicine have been used successfully in selected cases. All of these agents have potentially serious side effects.

ULCERATIVE LESIONS

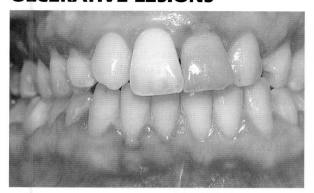

Fig. 44-1. Persistent ulcers on marginal and attached gingiva in a patient with **major aphthous.**

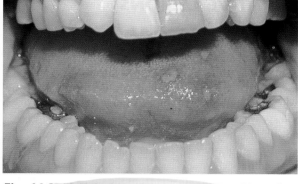

Fig. 44-2. Multiple tongue ulcers in patient with **major aphthous.**

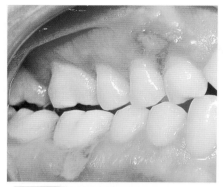

Fig. 44-3. Painful **major aphthous** of the gingiva.

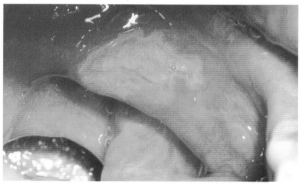

Fig. 44-4. Large irregular ulcer of the soft palate; same patient with **major aphthous** as in Figs. 44-1 through 44-3

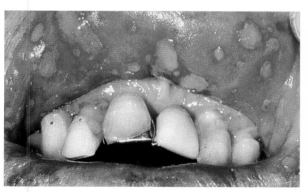

Fig. 44-5. Multiple **herpetiform ulcerations** of the labial mucosa. (Courtesy Dr Geza Terezhalmy)

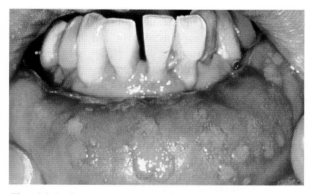

Fig. 44-6. Coalescing **herpetiform ulcerations;** same patient as in Fig. 44-5. (Courtesy Dr Geza Terezhalmy)

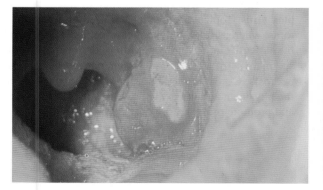

Fig. 44-7. Young male with tonsillar ulceration of **Behçet's syndrome.** (Courtesy Dr Geza Terezhalmy)

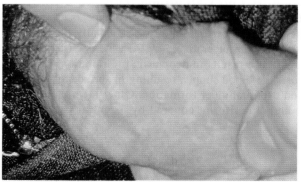

Fig. 44-8. Multiple genital ulcers in the same patient as seen in Fig. 44-7; **Behçet's syndrome.** (Courtesy Dr Geza Terezhalmy)

Sexually Related and Infectious Conditions

Appendix I

Rx Abbreviations

Appendix I
Rx ABBREVIATIONS

ABBREVIATION	ENGLISH	LATIN DERIVATIVE
ad lib	at pleasure	ad libitium
a.c.	before meals	ante cibum
p.c.	after meals	post cibum
aq.	water	aqua
d.	a day, daily	dies
b.i.d.	twice a day	bis in die
t.i.d.	three times a day	ter in die
q.i.d.	four times a day	quater in die
h.	hour	hora
h.s.	at bedtime	hora somni
q.h.	every hour	quaque hora
q.3h.	every three hours	quaque tertia hora
q.4h.	every four hours	quaque quarta hora
q.6h.	every six hours	quaque sexta hora
n.r.	do not repeat	non repetatur
p.r.n.	as needed	pro re nata
stat.	immediately	statim
Sig.	label	signetur
c.	with	cum
gtt.	drops	guttae
tab	tablet	tabella
caps.	capsule	capsula
q.d.	every day	quaque die

Appendix II

Therapeutic Protocols

ANALGESICS

TREATMENT RATIONALE:
For the relief of the symptoms of mild to moderate pain associated with oral conditions.

Rx   Acetaminophen Tylenol® 325 mg (McNeil)
Tylenol® 325 mg (McNeil)

Disp.: 100 Tablets

Sig: Take 2 tables q.4 h. p.r.n. pain not to exceed 12 tabs in 24 hours.

Rx   Acetylsalicylic Acid
Bayer Aspirin® 325 mg (Glenbrook)

Disp.: 100 Tablets

Sig: Take 2 tablets q.4 h. p.r.n. pain.

Rx   Ibuprofen
Motrin® 400 mg (Upjohn)

Disp.: 100 Tablets

Sig: Take 2 tablets q.4 h. p.r.n. pain.

Rx   Naproxen
Naprosyn® 375mg (Syntex)

Disp.: 50 Tablets

Sig: Take 2 tablets t.i.d. p.r.n. pain.

Rx   Acetaminophen with Codeine 30 mg
Tylenol with Codeine No.3 ® Tablets (McNeil Pharm)

Disp.: 30 Tablets

Sig: Take 2 tablets q.4 h. p.r.n. pain.

Rx   Aspirin with Codeine 30 mg
Empirin with Codeine No.3 ® Tablets (Burroughs Wellcome)

Disp.: 30 Tablets

Sig: Take 2 tablets q.4 h. p.r.n. pain.

ANALGESICS

Rx   Aspirin 325 mg, Butalbital 50 mg, Caffiene 40 mg
Fiorinal tabs ® (Sandoz)

Disp.: 40 Tablets

Sig: Take 1 to 2 tablets q.4 h. p.r.n. pain.

Rx   Dihydrocodeine bitartrate 16 mg, Aspirin 356.4 mg, Caffeine 30 mg
Synalgos-DC® Capsules (Wyeth)

Disp.: 40 Tablets

Sig: Take 1 to 2 tablets q.4 h. p.r.n. pain.

Rx   Oxycodone HCl 5 mg, Acetaminophen 325 mg
Percocet® Tablets (Dupont)

Disp.: 25 Tablets

Sig: Take 1 tablet q.4 h. p.r.n. pain.

Rx   Oxycodone HCl 4.5 mg, Oxycodone Terephthalate 0.38 mg, Aspirin 325 mg
Percodan® Tablets (Dupont)

Disp.: 25 Tablets

Sig: Take 1 tablet q.4 h. p.r.n. pain.

Rx   Meperidine HCl 50 mg, Promethazine HCl 25 mg
Mepergan Fortis ® Capsules (Wyeth)

Disp.: 25 Tablets

Sig: Take 1 tablet q.4 to 6 h. p.r.n. pain.

Rx   Hydrocodone bitartrate 5 mg, Acetaminophen 500 mg
Lortab® 5 Tablets (Russ)

Disp: 30 Tablets

Sig: Take 1 tablet q.4 h. p.r.n. pain.

Appendix II
THERAPEUTIC PROTOCOLS

FLUORIDE THERAPY

TREATMENT RATIONALE:
To prevent dental caries in susceptible patients.

Rx Stannous fluoride 0.4%

Disp.: 4.3 fl oz

Sig: Apply 5 to 10 drops in a carrier and place carrier on teeth daily for 5 minutes.

Rx Oral fluoride
0.125 mg Luride ® per drop (ColgateHoyt)

Disp.: 60 ml bottle with dropper

Sig: Apply 2 drops per day* (Birth to 2 years)
Apply 4 drops per day* (2 to 3 years)
Apply 8 drops per day* (3 to 12 years)
*in the mouth of the child.

TOPICAL ORAL ANESTHETICS

TREATMENT RATIONALE:
Relief of the symptoms associated with minor irritations of the mouth.

Rx Diphenhydramine HCl
Benadryl ® elixir 12.5 mg/5 ml (Parke-Davis)

Disp.: 4 fl oz

Sig: Rinse with 1 tablespoon a.c. and p.r.n. pain.

Rx Benadryl ® elixir 12.5 mg/5 ml (Parke-Davis) and Kaopectate ® (Upjohn), 50% mixture by volume

Disp.: 4 fl oz of each, mix equal parts

Sig: Rinse with 1 tablespoon for 2 minutes a.c. and p.r.n. pain.

Rx Lidocaine HCl
2% Xylocaine ® viscous solution (Astra)

Disp.: 4 fl oz

Sig: Rinse with 1 teaspoon a.c. and p.r.n. pain. Expectorate after rinsing.

Rx Orabase with Benzocaine (Colgate-Hoyt)

Disp.: 5 gm (15 gm)

Sig: Apply to affected area a.c. and p.r.n. pain.

ANTIANXIETY AGENTS

TREATMENT RATIONALE:
For the management and short-term relief of the symptoms of anxiety.

Rx Chlordiazepoxide
    Librium ® 10 mg (Roche)

Disp.: 20 Tablets

Sig: Take 1 tablet twice daily.

Rx Diazepam
    Valium ® 5 mg (Roche)

Disp.: 20 Tablets

Sig: Take 1 tablet 2-3 times daily, and 1 tablet 1 hour before dental appointments.

Rx Alpraxolam
    Xanax ® 0.25 mg (Upjohn)

Disp.: 20 Tablets

Sig: Take 1 tablet twice daily.

Rx Buspirone
    Buspar ® 5 mg (Mead Johnson)

Disp.: 20 Tablets

Sig: Take 1 tablet twice daily.

NUTRIENT DEFICIENCY THERAPY

TREATMENT RATIONALE:
To replace deficient nutrients necessary for homeostasis.

Rx Ferrous sulfate 250 mg

Disp.: 100 Tablets

Sig: Take 1 tablet t.i.d. for 1 month, then re-assess patient's hemoglobin.

Rx Folic acid 0.4 mg

Disp.: 30 Tablets

Sig: Take 1 tablet daily for 1 month, then re-assess patient's folic acid level.*

***Caution:** Medical supervision is advised.

Rx Water soluble bioflavinoids 200 mg
    with ascorbic acid 200 mg
    Peridin-C ® 400 mg (Beutlich)

Disp.: 100 Tablets

Sig: Take 1 tablet t.i.d. for 2 weeks.

ANTIHISTAMINES

TREATMENT RATIONALE:
To reduce the effects of histamine-mediated hypersensitivity and temporary relief of the symptoms associated with minor oral irritations.

Rx   Diphenhydramine HCl
             Benadryl ® 25 mg (Parke-Davis)

Disp.:   40 Tablets

Sig: Take 1 tablet every 6 hours as needed.

Rx   Brompheniramine Maleate HCl
             Dimetane ® 4 mg (Robins)

Disp.:   40 Tablets

Sig: Take 1 or 2 tablets every 6 hours as needed.

Rx   Phenylpropanolamine HCl 25 mg and
             Brompheniramine Maleate HCl 4 mg
             Dimetapp ® (Robins)

Disp.:   40 Tablets

Sig: Take 1 tablet q.4 h. as needed.

Rx   Terfenadine
             Seldane ® 60 mg (Merrell Dow)

Disp.:   30 Tablets

Sig: Take 1 tablet twice a day.

Rx   Astemizole
             Hismanal ® 10 mg (Janssen)

Disp: 25 Tablets

Sig: Take 1 tablet once a day.

SALIVA SUBSTITUTE

TREATMENT RATIONALE:
For the relief of a dry mouth.

Rx   Carboxymethyl cellulose 0.5% aqueous solution.

Disp.:   8 fl oz

Sig: Use as a rinse p.r.n.

Rx   Moi-stir ® (Kingswood)

Disp.:   120 ml with pump spray

Sig: Use as a rinse p.r.n.

Rx   Xerolube ® (Scherer)

Disp.:   180 ml with pump spray

Sig: Use as a rinse p.r.n.

Rx   Salivart ® (Westport Pharm)

Disp.:   75 ml with pump spray

Sig: Use as a rinse p.r.n.

ANTI-FUNGAL THERAPY

TREATMENT RATIONALE:
To eliminate pathogenic fungal organisms and to reestablish the normal oral flora.

Rx Nystatin vaginal tablets
Nilstat ®100,000 I.U. (Lederle)

Disp.: 90 Tablets

Sig: Dissolve 1 tablet as a lozenge 5 times daily for 14 consecutive days.

Note: Remove denture(s) if applicable.

Rx Clotrimazole
Mycelex Troches ® 10 mg (Miles Pharm)

Disp.: 60 Tablets

Sig: Dissolve 1 tablet as a lozenge 5 times daily for 14 consecutive days.

Note: Remove denture(s) if applicable.

Rx Ketoconazole
Nizoral ® 200 mg (Janssen Pharm)

Disp.: 14 Tablets

Sig: Take 1 tablet daily for 2 weeks.

Rx Nystatin
Mycostatin Pastilles ® 200,000 U (Squibb)

Disp.: 60 Tablets

Sig: Dissolve 1 pastille in mouth 4 times daily as a lozenge for 14 consecutive days.

Note: Remove denture(s) if applicable.

Rx Nystatin topical powder
Mycostatin ® topical powder 100,000 I.U. (Squibb)

Disp.: 15 gm squeeze bottle

Sig: Apply liberally to tissue side of clean denture p.c. Soak the clean denture in a suspension of 1 teaspoon of powder and 8 oz. of water over night.

ANTI-FUNGAL THERAPY

Rx Nystatin ointment
Mycostatin ointment ® 100,000 I.U. (Squibb)

Disp.: 15 gm (30 gm) tube

Sig: Apply liberally to affected area 4 to 6 times daily.

Rx Nystatin-neomycin sulfate-gramicidin-triamcinolone acetomide
Tri-Statin ® (Rugby)

Disp.: 15 gm (30, 60 gm) tube

Sig: Apply liberally to affected area 3 to 4 times daily.

ANTI-VIRAL THERAPY

TREATMENT RATIONALE:
To prevent and/or treat oral herpetic infections.

Rx Acyclovir ointment
5% Zovirax ® (Burroughs Wellcome)

Disp.: 15 gm

Sig: Apply to oral lesions with a cotton tip applicator 6 times a day.

Note: Treatment should begin during the early (prodromal) stage of the recurrence.

Rx Acyclovir
Zovirax ® 200 mg (Burroughs Wellcome)

Disp.: 50 Capsules

Sig: 1 capsule q.4.h. for 5 to 10 days.

Note: Treatment should begin during the early stage of the recurrence in the immunosuppressed patient.

Rx L-Lysine
Enisyl ® 500 mg (Person & Covey)

Disp.: 100 Tablets

Sig: Take 4 tablets q.4.h. until symptoms subside.

Note: Treatment should begin during the early stage of the recurrence.

SEDATIVE/HYPNOTICS

TREATMENT RATIONALE:
To produce a "sleep-like" state for the effective management of an oral disease or condition.

Rx   Triazolam
Halcion ® 0.25 mg (Upjohn)

Disp.: 30 Tablets

Sig: Take 1 tablet h.s.

Rx   Flurazepam
Dalmane ®15 mg (Roche)

Disp.: 30 Tablets

Sig: Take 1 tablet h.s.

Rx   Temazepam
Restoril ® 15 mg (Sandoz)

Disp.: 30 Tablets

Sig: Take 1 tablet h.s.

Rx   Chloral hydrate
Noctec ® 500 mg/ 5 ml (Squibb)

Disp.: 1 pint

Sig: Take 1 teaspoon before bedtime or 30 minutes before surgery.

ANTIBIOTIC THERAPY

TREATMENT RATIONALE:
To eliminate pathogenic bacterial organisms that cause oral infection.

Rx   Phenoxymethyl Penicillin
Penicillin V 500 mg Tablets

Disp.: 40 Tabs

Sig: Take 2 tablets immediately and then 1 tab q.6 h. 1 hour before meals.

Rx   Penicillin V Potassium liquid
Penicillin VK liquid 125 mg/5 ml

Disp.: 200 ml

Sig: Child should take 1 teaspoonful q.6 h.

Rx   Amoxicillin
Amoxil ® 500 mg (Beecham Labs)

Disp.: 40 Tabs

Sig: Take 1 500 mg tablet q.8 h.

Rx   Dicloxacillin Sodium
Dynapen ® 500 mg (Bristol)

Disp.: 40 Tabs

Sig: Take 1 500 mg tablet q.8 h.

Note: For penicillinase-resistant infection.

Rx   Trimethoprim 80 mg and
Sulfamethoxazole 400 mg
Bactrim ® (Roche)

Disp.: 40 Tabs

Sig: Take 1 tablet q.12 h.

Note: For infections involving Escherichia coli, Hemophilus influenzae, Klebsiella and Enterobacter species.

ANTIBIOTIC THERAPY

Rx Metronidazole
Flagyl ® 500 mg (Searle)

Disp.: 40 Tabs

Sig: Take 2 tablets immediately, then 1 tablet q.6 h. until gone.

Note: For a febrile patient with acute necrotizing ulcerative gingivitis involving anaerobic bacteria.

Rx Erythromycin ethylsuccinate 400
EES ® 400 mg (Abbott)

Disp.: 56 Tabs

Sig: Take 1 400 mg tablet q.6 h. Continue for 7 days.

Rx Tetracycline HCl
Achromycin V ® 250 mg (Lederle)

Disp.: 56 Tabs

Sig: Take 1 tablet q.i.d. Continue for 7 days.

Rx Cephalexin
Keflex ® 250 mg (Dista)

Disp.: 56 Tabs

Sig: Take 2 tablets q.6 h. Continue for 7 days.

BACTERIAL ENDOCARDITIS PROPHYLAXIS

Rx Clindamycin
Disp: By weight

Sig: 10 mg/kg 1hr prior to dental treatment, followed by half the original dose 6 hr after the initial loading dose

Note: For the prevention of infective endocarditis in children allergic to penicillins.

ANTIBIOTIC THERAPY – BACTERIAL ENDOCARDITIS PROPHYLAXIS

TREATMENT RATIONALE:
To prevent bacterial endocarditis in patients with rheumatic, congenital, or other acquired valvular heart disease who are undergoing dental procedures.

Rx Amoxicillin, 500 mg

Disp.: 9 tabs (4.5 grams)

Sig: Take 6 tabs (3 g), orally 1hr before dental procedure, then 1.5 g 6 hr after the initial dose.

Note: Standard regimen for the prevention of bacterial endocarditis in adults and children > 66 lbs; (30 kg)

Rx Amoxicillin, 250 mg

Disp.: By weight

Sig: Take 50 mg/kg, orally, 1hr before dental treatment, followed by half the original dose 6 hr after the original dose.

Note: Standard regimen for the prevention of infective endocarditis in children < 66 lbs (30 kg). The following weight ranges may also be used for the initial pediatric dose of amoxicillin < 15kg, 750 mg; 15 to 30 kg, 1500 mg; and > 30 kg, 3000 mg.

Rx Erythromycin* ethylsuccinate, 400 mg

Disp.: 3 Tabs

Sig: Take 2 tabs orally, 2 hr before dental treatment, followed by half the original dose 6 hr after the initial loading dose.

OR

Rx Clindamycin, 150 mg

Disp.: 3 Tabs

Sig: Take 2 tabs orally, 1hr before dental treatment, followed by half the original dose 6 hr after the initial loading dose.

Note: For patients allergic to penicillin.

* Note: Differences in absorption and bio-availability require changes in dosing when using different forms of erythromycin.

ANTIBIOTIC THERAPY – BACTERIAL ENDOCARDITIS PROPHYLAXIS HIGH RISK PROTOCOL – ADULT

Rx   Ampicillin

Disp.: 2 g

Sig: 2 g IM or IV 30 min prior to dental treatment.

PLUS

Rx   Gentamycin

Disp.: By weight

Sig: 1.5 mg/kg IM or IV 30 min prior to dental treatment

THEN

1.5 g, Amoxicillin, orally 6 hr after initial dose

OR

The parenteral regimen may be repeated 6 hr after initial dose

Note: For maximum protection against bacterial endocarditis in adults at risk.

ANTIBIOTIC THERAPY – BACTERIAL ENDOCARDITIS PROPHYLAXIS HIGH RISK PROTOCOL – CHILD

Rx   Ampicillin

Disp.: By weight

Sig: 50 mg/kg IM or IV 30 min prior to dental treatment

PLUS

Rx   Gentamycin

Disp.: By weight

Sig: 2 mg/kg IM or IV 30 min prior to dental treatment

THEN

One half the initial dose 6 hr later

Note: For prevention of bacterial endocarditis in children under 66 lbs (30 kg).

ALTERNATIVE INTRAVENOUS REGIMEN – ADULT

Rx   Vancomycin
Vancocin (Lilly) in parenteral solution

Disp.: 1g

Sig: Slowly administer 1g over 1 hr intravenously beginning 1 hr prior to dental procedure.

Note: For prevention of bacterial endocarditis in penicillin-allergic, high-risk adult patients undergoing dental procedures.

ALTERNATIVE INTRAVENOUS REGIMEN – CHILD

Rx   Vancomycin
Vancocin (Lilly) in parental solution

Disp.: By weight

Sig: 20 mg/kg IV given slowly over 1 hr, beginning 1 hr prior to dental procedure

Note: For prevention of bacterial endocarditis in penicillin-allergic, high-risk children undergoing dental procedures.

Appendix III

**Guide to Diagnosis
and Management of
Common Oral Lesions**

Appendix III
GUIDE TO DIAGNOSIS AND MANAGEMENT OF COMMON ORAL LESIONS
WHITE LESIONS

Disease	Age	Sex	Race/ Ethnicity	Clinical Characteristics	Treatment
Fordyce's granules	Any	M–F	Any	Whitish-yellow granules clustered in plaques located on buccal mucosa (bilaterally), labial mucosa, retromolar pad, lip, attached gingiva, tongue, and frenum. Lesions are nontender, rough to palpation, and do not rub off. Onset after puberty; persists for life.	None required.
Linea alba buccalis	Any	M–F	Any	White wavy line of varying length located on buccal mucosa, bilaterally. Lesions are nontender, smooth to palpation, and do not rub off. Variable onset; persists with oral habits.	Eliminate bruxism and clenching.
Leukoedema	Any	M–F	Melanoderms	Grayish-white patch of variable size located on buccal mucosa (bilaterally), labial mucosa, and soft palate. Lesions are nontender, smooth to palpation and disappear when the mucosa is stretched. Leukoedema becomes more evident with increasing age.	None required.
Morsicatio buccarum	Any	M–F	Any	Asymmetric white plaque located on buccal mucosa and labial mucosa, often bilaterally. Lesions are nontender, rough to palpation, and peel slightly when rubbed. Variable onset; persists with cheek or lip biting habit.	Eliminate cheek/ lip chewing habit.
White sponge nevus	Any	M–F	Any	Solitary or confluent raised white plaques that may appear on buccal mucosa, labial mucosa, alveolar ridge, floor of the mouth, and/or soft palate. Lesions are nontender, rough to palpation, and do not rub off. Onset at birth; persists for life.	None required.
Traumatic white lesions	Any	M–F	Any	White surface slough (eschar) usually located on the less-keratinized alveolar mucosa. Palate common for food "burns". Lesions are tender to palpation and rub off leaving a raw or bleeding surface. Onset within hours of trauma; regression in 1 to 2 weeks.	Eliminate irritant; topical anesthetics and analgesics.
Leukoplakia	45 – 65	2:1 (M:F)	Any	White patch that varies in size, homogeneity, and texture. High risk locations include floor of the mouth, ventral tongue, lateral tongue, and uvulo-palatal complex. Lesions do not rub off and usually are nontender. Onset occurs after prolonged contact with an inducing agent; persists as long as the inducing agent is present.	Biopsy and histologic examination. Close follow-up mandatory.
Cigarette keratosis	Elderly	M	Any	White pebbly circular patches located on upper and lower lips (kissing lesions). Keratoses are firm, nontender, and do not rub off. Onset in conjunction with a prolonged cigarette smoking habit; persists with habit.	Use filtered cigarettes, or stop smoking. Biopsy if lesion becomes ulcerated or indurated.

GUIDE TO DIAGNOSIS AND MANAGEMENT OF COMMON ORAL LESIONS
WHITE LESIONS

Disease	Age	Sex	Race/ Ethnicity	Clinical Characteristics	Treatment
Nicotine stomatitis	40 – 70	M	Any	White cobblestoned papules located on hard palate, excluding the anterior third. Papules have red centers, are nontender, and do not rub off. Onset is variable to degree of smoking; lesions are long-standing.	Stop pipe/ cigar/reverse smoking habit.
Snuff dipper's patch	Teenage and adult	M	Any	Corrugated whitish-yellow patch located on mucobuccal fold, most prominent unilaterally. Patch is rough, nontender and does not rub off. Long-standing habit precedes lesion; patch persists with continuation of habit.	Discontinue tobacco use. Biopsy if change in color, or if lesion becomes ulcerated or indurated.
Verrucous carcinoma	Over 60	M	Any	Papulonodular whitish-red mass located on buccal mucosa, alveolar ridge, gingiva. Lesion is firm, nontender, rough to palpation, and does not rub off. Long-standing tobacco habit precedes onset; lesion enlarges unless treated.	Biopsy to confirm diagnosis, then surgical excision. AVOID RADIATION THERAPY.
Squamous cell carcinoma	(see Red and/or Red/White Lesions)				

GUIDE TO DIAGNOSIS AND MANAGEMENT OF COMMON ORAL LESIONS
RED LESIONS

Disease	Age	Sex	Race/ Ethnicity	Clinical Characteristics	Treatment
Purpura	Any	M–F	Any	Red spot or patch consisting of extravasated blood that onsets soon after trauma. Lesions do not blanch upon diascopy and size varies (petechiae < ecchymosis < hematoma). Petechiae common on soft palate; other purpurae typically occur on buccal/labial mucosa, depending on site at which blood pools. Lesions fade away.	Eliminate underlying problem.
Varicosity	Over 55	F	Any	Reddish-purple papule or nodule located on ventral tongue, lip, or labial mucosa. Lesions are asymptomatic and blanch upon diascopy. Varicosities increase in size and number with increasing age and are persistent.	None necessary. Surgery for esthetics.
Thrombus	Over 30	M–F	Any	Red to blue-purple nodule located on labial mucosa, lip, or tongue. Lesions are firm and may be tender to palpation. Onset after traumatic bleed; lesion is diascopy negative and persists until treatment. Occasionally thrombi will spontaneously regress.	Surgical removal and histologic examination, if persistent or symptomatic.
Hemangioma	Child – adolescent	F	Any	Red to purple, soft, smooth-surfaced or multinodular exophytic mass located on dorsal tongue, buccal mucosa, or gingiva. Lesions are diascopy positive. Onset early in life; persists until treated. Occasionally hemangiomas will spontaneously regress.	If present since youth, no functional disability, and no changes in size, shape, or color, no treatment is necessary, otherwise, surgery/ histologic exam.
Hereditary hemorrhagic telangiectasia	Post-puberty	M–F	Any	Multifocal red macules located on palms, fingers, nail beds, face, neck, conjunctiva, nasal septum, lips, tongue, hard palate, and gingiva. Lesions are present at birth, become more visible at puberty, and increase in number with age. Telangiectasias lack central pulsation, blanch upon diascopy, and if they rupture severe bleeding may result.	None required. Monitor for hemorrhage and/or anemia.
Sturge-Weber syndrome	Birth	M–F	Any	Syndrome associated with seizures, mental deficits, gyriform calcifications, and a red to purple flat or slightly raised facial hemangioma. Vascular lesion often affects lips, labial/buccal mucosa, gingiva along branches of trigeminal nerve. Abnormal oral enlargements may be concurrent.	None required. Elective surgery for esthetics.
Kaposi's sarcoma	20-45 and over 60	M	Jewish, Mediterranean or HIV-infected	Asymptomatic red macule of mucocutaneous structures that enlarges and becomes raised and then darkens in color. Advanced lesions are red-blue-violet nodules that ulcerate and cause pain. The hard palate, gingiva, and buccal mucosa are the most common oral locations.	Palliative, consisting of radiation therapy, laser surgery, chemotherapy, or a combination thereof.

GUIDE TO DIAGNOSIS AND MANAGEMENT OF COMMON ORAL LESIONS
RED AND RED/WHITE LESIONS

Disease	Age	Sex	Race/ Ethnicity	Clinical Characteristics	Treatment
Erythroplakia	Over 50	M>F	Any	Red patch of variable size located on any oral mucosal site. High risk areas include floor of the mouth, soft palate-retromolar trigone, lateral border of tongue. Erythroplakias do not rub off and are usually asymptomatic. Lesions onset after prolonged contact with carcinogens; duration is variable. Regression is rare.	Biopsy and histologic examination. Close follow-up.
Erythroleukoplakia & speckled erythroplakia	Over 50	M	Any	Red patch with multiple foci of white. Nontender, do not rub off, often superficially infected with candida. Common locations include lateral tongue, buccal mucosa, soft palate, and floor of the mouth. Onset after prolonged exposure to carcinogens. Regression unlikely even if inducing agent is removed.	Biopsy and histologic examination. Examine for candidiasis. Close follow-up.
Squamous cell carcinoma	Over 50	2:1 M:F	Any	Red, red/white, or ulcer commonly located on lateral tongue, ventral tongue, oropharynx, floor of the mouth, gingiva, buccal mucosa, or lip. Carcinoma often asymptomatic until it becomes large, indurated, or ulcerated. Onset after prolonged exposure to carcinogens. Persistence results in metastasis, usually apparent as painless, firm, matted, fixed lymph nodes.	Biopsy and histologic examination. Complete surgical removal, radiation therapy, or chemotherapy. Close follow-up.
Lichen planus	Over 40	F	Any	Purple, polygonal, pruritic papules on flexor surfaces of skin; occasionally finger nails are affected. Intraoral lesions are often symptomatic and consist of white linear papules, reddish, patches and ulcerated regions of mucosa. Affected surfaces are often bilateral. Most common locations include buccal mucosa, tongue, lips, palate, gingiva, and the floor of the mouth. Lesions onset with stress; persist for many years with periods of remission and exacerbation.	Rest, anxiolytics, topical corticosteroids, close follow-up for occasional malignant transformation in the erosive type.
Electrogalvanic white lesion	Over 30	F	Any	Reddish-white patches that resemble lichen planus located on buccal mucosa adjacent to metallic restorations. Lesions do not rub off and are usually tender or cause a burning sensation. Onset after weeks to years of exposure to metallic restoration; duration is variable depending on the persistence of the allergen.	Replace metallic restoration or clasp that is causing the hypersensitive response.
Lupus erythematosus	Over 40	F	Any	Reddish butterfly rash on bridge of nose. Maculo-papular eruption with atrophic central areas may involve the lower lip, buccal mucosa, tongue and palate. Intraoral lesions invariably have red and white radiating lines emanating from the lesion. Lesions do not rub off, but are tender to palpation. Onset often after acute sun exposure. Lesions persist and require drug treatment.	Topical and systemic steroids; antimalarials in conjunction with adequate medical treatment.

Appendix III

GUIDE TO DIAGNOSIS AND MANAGEMENT OF COMMON ORAL LESIONS
RED AND RED/WHITE LESIONS

Disease	Age	Sex	Race/ Ethnicity	Clinical Characteristics	Treatment
Lichenoid & lupus-like drug eruption	Adult	M–F	Any	Red-white patches that resemble lichen planus and lupus. Often the lesions are atrophic or ulcerated centrally. Buccal mucosa, bilaterally, is the most common site. Onset is variable and may be weeks or years after an allergic medication is begun. Regression occurs when the offending drug is eliminated.	Withdraw offending drug and substitute medication.
Candidiasis	Newborns, adults	M–F	Any	Variable appearance; white curds, red patches, white patches with red margins. Any oral soft tissue site is susceptible; however, the attached gingiva is rarely affected. Onset is often coincident with neutropenia, and/or immune suppression. Lesions persist until adequate antifungal therapy is provided.	Antifungal therapy. Eliminate diabetes, endo-crinopathy, immune-suppression.

GUIDE TO DIAGNOSIS AND MANAGEMENT OF COMMON ORAL LESIONS
PIGMENTED LESIONS

Disease	Age	Sex	Race/ Ethnicity	Clinical Characteristics	Treatment
Melanoplakia	Any	M–F	Melanoderms	Generalized constant dark patch located on attached gingiva and buccal mucosa. Pigmentation varies from light brown to dark brown and is often diffuse, curvilinear, asymptomatic, and does not rub off. Melanoplakia present at birth and persists for life.	None required.
Tattoo	Teenagers adults	M–F	Any	Amalgam tattoo is the most common type of intraoral tattoo. Appears as a blue-black macule on gingiva, edentulous ridge, vestibule, palate, or buccal mucosa. Radiographs may demonstrate radiopaque foci. Lesions are asymptomatic, do not blanch, and persist for life.	None required.
Ephelis	Any	M–F	Light-skinned persons	Light to dark brown macule that appears on facial skin, extremities, or lip following sun exposure. Ephelides are initially small but may enlarge and coalesce. Lesions are nontender and do not blanch or rub off.	None required.
Smoker's melanosis	Older adult	M–F	Any	Diffuse brown patch of several centimeters, usually on posterior buccal mucosa and soft palate. History of heavy tobacco smoking precedes development of the lesion. Features may decrease with discontinuation of the habit. Melanosis is asymptomatic and nonpalpable.	Diminish or stop smoking.
Oral melanotic macule	25 – 45	Slight male predilection	Any	Asymptomatic brown to black macule usually located on lower lip near midline; also occurs on palate, buccal mucosa, and gingiva. Onset is post-inflammatory and the lesion persists until treatment.	Biopsy and histologic examination to rule out other similar appearing pigmented lesions.
Nevus	Any	F	Any	Nevi are highly variable in appearance. They may be pink, blue, brown, or black, but do not blanch upon diascopy. They usually appear as a bluish or brownish smooth-surfaced papule located on the palate. Other common sites include the buccal mucosa, face, neck, and trunk. Many lesions are present at birth. They increase in size and number with increased age.	Excisional biopsy and histologic examination.
Melanoma	25 – 60	M	Caucasians, especially light-skinned persons	Painless, slightly raised plaque or patch that has multiple colors, especially foci of brown, black, gray, or red. Ill-defined margins, satellite lesions, and inflammatory borders are characteristic. They are usually located on maxillary alveolar ridge, palate, anterior gingiva, and labial mucosa. 30% arise from pre-existing pigmentations. A recent change in size, shape, or color is particularly ominous.	Excisional biopsy, surgical removal, and referral for complete medical work-up to rule out metastasis.

GUIDE TO DIAGNOSIS AND MANAGEMENT OF COMMON ORAL LESIONS
PIGMENTED LESIONS

Disease	Age	Sex	Race/ Ethnicity	Clinical Characteristics	Treatment
Peutz-Jeghers syndrome	Child, young adult	M–F	Any	Multiple, asymptomatic melanotic oval macules, prominently located on the skin of the palmar/ plantar surfaces of the hands and feet, around the eyes, nose, mouth, lips, and perineum. Intraorally, brown discolorations occur on the buccal mucosa, labial mucosa, and gingiva. Lesions do not increase in size, but cutaneous lesions often fade with age; mucosal pigmentation persists for life. Colickly intestinal symptoms are probable.	Oral: none required. Gastro-intestinal evaluation and genetic counseling.
Addison's disease	Adult	M–F	Any	Diffuse intraoral hypermelanotic patches occuring in conjunction with bronzing of the skin, especially of the knuckles, elbows, and palmar creases. Patches are nontender, nonraised, and variable in shape. The buccal mucosa and gingiva are most commonly affected. Onset of the disorder is insidious and associated with adrenal gland hypofunction. Patient may complain of gastrointestinal symptoms and fatigue.	Systemic cortico-steroids.
Heavy metal pigmentation	Adult	M–F	Any	Blue-black linear pigmentation of marginal gingiva, prominently viewed along anterior gingiva. Spotty gray macules may be apparent on buccal mucosa. Neuralgic symptoms, headache, hypersalivation are common. Argyria: blue-gray skin pigmentation, especially in sun-exposed areas.	Terminate exposure to heavy metal, medical referral. Oral lesions require no treatment.

GUIDE TO DIAGNOSIS AND MANAGEMENT OF COMMON ORAL LESIONS
VESICULOBULLOUS DISEASES

Disease	Age	Sex	Race/ Ethnicity	Clinical Characteristics	Treatment
Primary herpetic gingivostomatitis	Infant, child, young adult	M–F	Any	Multiple vesicles that rupture, coalesce, and form ulcers of the lip, buccal and labial mucosa, gingiva, palate, and tongue. Ulcers are painful and initially are small, yellow, and have red inflammatory borders, Onset is rapid, several days after contact with person harboring the virus. Lesions persist for 12 to 20 days.	Fluids, antipyretics, antibiotics to prevent secondary infection, oral anesthetic rinses, analgesics.
Recurrent herpes simplex	Adult	M–F	Any	Multiple small vesicles that rupture and ulcerate. These lesions occur repeatedly at same site, usually the lip, hard palate, and attached gingiva. Onset is rapid; preceded by prodromal burning or tingling. Duration is 5 to 12 days. Heals spontaneously.	Bioflavanoids, sunscreens (lip), lysine. Acyclovir in severe cases or when immune-suppressed.
Herpangina	Child, young adult	M–F	Any	Light gray papillary vesicles that rupture forming multiple discrete shallow ulcers. Lesions have erythematous border and are limited to anterior pillars, soft palate, uvula, and tonsils. Pharyngitis, headache, fever, and lymphadenitis are often concurrent. Lesions heal spontaneously within 1 to 2 weeks.	Palliative, heals spontaneously.
Chicken pox	Child	M–F	Any	Vesicles on skin and face that after rupturing resemble a "dew drop." Intraorally ulcers may be seen on soft palate, buccal mucosa, and mucobuccal fold. Skin lesions crust over and heal with scar formation. Condition often accompanied by chills, fever nasopharyngitis, and malaise. Spontaneous healing occurs in 7 to 10 days.	Palliative, heals spontaneously. Avoid scratching to limit scar formation.
Herpes zoster	Over 55, over 35 in HIV+	M–F	Any	Unilateral vesicular and pustular eruptions that develop over 1 to 3 days. Lesions occur along dermatomes and especially along the trigeminal nerve tract. Lesions are vesicular, ulcerative, intensely painful and commonly affect the lip, tongue and buccal mucosa extending up to the midline. Neuralgia may persist after healing.	Palliative, heals spontaneously, acyclovir in severe cases or immunosup= pressed.
Hand-foot-and-mouth disease	Child, young adult	M–F	Any	Crops of multiple small yellowish ulcers that occur on palm and sole of hand and foot. Intraorally the tongue, hard palate, buccal and labial mucosa are affected. Total number of lesions may approach 100. Healing occurs spontaneously in about 10 days.	Palliative, heals spontaneously.
Allergic reactions immediate	Any	M–F	Any	Red swellings or wheals that occur periorally or on lips, buccal mucosa, gingiva, lips, and tongue. Contact with allergen usually precedes episode by a few minutes to hours. Warmth, tenseness, and itchiness are concurrent. Lesions regress if the allergen is withdrawn.	Remove allergen; antihistamines.

GUIDE TO DIAGNOSIS AND MANAGEMENT OF COMMON ORAL LESIONS
VESICULOBULLOUS DISEASES

Disease	Age	Sex	Race/ Ethnicity	Clinical Characteristics	Treatment
Allergic reactions delayed	Any	M–F	Any	Itchy erythematous lesions that may eventually ulcerate. May occur on any cutaneous or mucocutaneous surface. Intraorally the lips, gingiva, alveolar mucosa, tongue, and palate are affected. Erythema develops slowly over 24 to 48 hours. Fissuring and ulceration may result.	Remove allergen; cortico-steroids.
Erythema multiforme	Young adult	M	Any	Skin – target lesions. Oral – hemorrhagic crust of the lips; painful ulcerations of the tongue, buccal mucosa. Attached gingiva rarely affected. Headache, low-grade fever, and previous respiratory infection often precedes lesions.	Topical analgesics, antipyretics, fluids, cortico-steroids, antibiotics to prevent secondary infection.
Stevens-Johnson syndrome	Child, young adult	Slight preference for males	Any	Skin – target lesions. Eye – conjunctivitis. Genital – balanitis. Oral – hemorrhagic crust of the lips; painful ulcerations and weeping bullae of the tongue, buccal mucosa. Attached gingiva rarely affected. Stevens-Johnson syndrome is the fulminant form of erythema multiforme. Eating and swallowing often are impaired.	Topical analgesics, antipyretics, fluids, cortico-steroids, antibiotics to prevent secondary infection, hospitalization.
Pemphigus vulgaris	30 – 50	M–F	Light skinned persons, Jewish and Mediterranean persons	Multiple skin and mucosal bullae that rupture, hemorrhage, and crust. Lesions tend to recur in the same area, have circular or serpiginous borders, and tend to spread to adjacent areas. Nikolsky sign positive. Collapsed bullae is a common sign. Dehydration can occur if lesions are extensive.	Medical referral, systemic steroids, and oral topical steroids.
Benign mucous membrane pemphigoid	Over 50	2:1 F:M	Any	Bullae on skin folds, inguinal and abdominal areas. Corneal lesions can lead to scarring. Bullae often are hemorrhagic and persist for days then desquamate. Lesions occur on the gingiva, palate and buccal mucosa.	Oral topical steroids. Medical referral and systemic steroids if severe; rule out corneal involvement and internal malignancy.

GUIDE TO DIAGNOSIS AND MANAGEMENT OF COMMON ORAL LESIONS
ULCERATIVE LESIONS

Disease	Age	Sex	Race/ Ethnicity	Clinical Characteristics	Treatment
Traumatic ulcer	Any	M–F	Any	Symptomatic, yellow-gray ulcer of variable size and shape, depending on inducing agent. Ulcers are often depressed and usually oval in shape with erythematous border. Commonly located on labial and buccal mucosa, tongue at the borders, and hard palate. Duration is 1 to 2 weeks.	Palliative; remove traumatic influence.
Recurrent aphthous stomatitis	Young adult	F	Any	Small yellowish oval ulcer with red border, located on movable non-keratinized mucosa. Common sites include labial mucosa, buccal mucosa, floor of the mouth, tongue, and occasionally soft palate. Ulcers are tender and may be associated with a tender lymph node. Lesions onset rapidly and disappear in 10 to 14 days without scar formation.	Spontaneous healing in 10 to 14 days. If acute symptoms or recurrently symptomatic, topical anesthetics, coagulating agents, or topical steroids may be used.
Pseudoaphthous ulcer	25 – 50	F	Any	Depressed yellowish round-oval ulcer located on movable non-keratinized mucosa. Common sites include labial mucosa, buccal mucosa, floor of the mouth, tongue, and occasionally soft palate. Tongue may demonstrate atrophied papillae. Ulcers are tender, onset during deficiency state and disappear with replacement therapy within 20 days.	Evaluate for deficiency state. If patient is deficient, then nutritional supplements (i.e. iron, B-12, folate) are recommended. Gluten abstinence may be required.
Major aphthous stomatitis	Young adult	F	Any	Asymmetric unilateral ulcer with necrotic and depressed center. Ulcers have a red inflammatory border and are extremely painful. Located on soft palate, tonsillar fauces, labial mucosa, buccal mucosa, tongue; may extend onto attached gingiva. Rapid onset. Underlying tissue is often destroyed. Lesions heal in 15 to 30 days with scar formation. Recurrences are common.	Spontaneous healing, sometimes with scar formation. Topical anesthetics, topical steroids, stress management, identify allergens.

GUIDE TO DIAGNOSIS AND MANAGEMENT OF COMMON ORAL LESIONS
ULCERATIVE LESIONS

Disease	Age	Sex	Race/ Ethnicity	Clinical Characteristics	Treatment
Herpetiform ulceration	20s	M	Any	Multiple pinhead-sized yellowish ulcers located on movable non-keratinized mucosa. Common sites include anterior tip of tongue, labial mucosa, and floor of the mouth. No vesicle formation. Ulcers are painful and may be associated with several tender lymph nodes. Lesions onset rapidly and disappear in 10 to 14 days without scar formation.	Tetracycline rinses.
Behçet's syndrome	20 – 30	3:1 (M:F)	Asian, Mediterranean, Anglo	Eye – conjunctivitis, iritis; Genital – ulcers; Oral – painful aphthous-like ulcers on labial and buccal mucosa; Skin – maculopapular rash and nodular eruptions. Oral ulcers are often an initial sign of the disease onset. Arthritis and gastrointestinal complaints may be concurrent. Recurrences, exacerbations, and remissions are likely.	Topical and systemic steroids.
Granulomatous ulcer (Tuberculosis, Histoplasmosis)	Older adult	M–F	Any	Asymptomatic, cobblestoned ulcer that usually occurs on dorsum of tongue, or labial commissure. Cervical lymphadenopathy and primary respiratory complaint often is concurrent. Onset of oral disease follows lung infection of several weeks to months duration. Oral ulcer may persist for months to years if underlying disease not treated.	Biopsy, histologic, examination. Tuberculosis – streptomycin and isoniazid. Histoplasmosis - Amphotericin B.
Squamous cell carcinoma	Over 50	2:1 M:F	Any	Nonpainful yellowish ulcer with red indurated borders commonly located on posterior third of the lateral border of tongue, ventral tongue, lips, and floor of the mouth. Associated features may nclude numbness, leukoplakia, erythroplakia, induration, fixation, fungation, and lymphadenopathy. Carcinoma has a slow onset and is often noticed after a recent increase in size.	Surgery, radiation therapy, and/or chemotherapy.
Chemo-therapeutic ulcer	15 to 30 and older adult	M–F	Any	Irregular ulcerations of the lips, labial and buccal mucosa, tongue, and palate. Red inflammatory border is often lacking. Hemorrhage is likely when ulcers are deeply situated. Lesions are extremely painful and usually limit mastication and swallowing. Onset during second week of chemotherapy. Secondary infection with oral microorganisms is likely.	Antimicrobial rinses to prevent secondary infection. Topical anesthetics, IV fluids.

Appendix IV

Self-Assessment Quiz

1. (Fig. 49-1) This soft tissue swelling was observed on the gingiva of a 7-month-old infant. The infant's mother states that during the past several days the lesion has slowly increased in size. Aspiration yielded a straw-colored fluid. This lesion is most likely a:

A. congenital epulis of the newborn
B. congenital lymphangioma
C. mucous retention phenomenon
D. gingival eruption cyst
E. traumatic hyperplasia

2. (Fig. 49-2) This dome-shaped papule on the ventral surface of the tongue is soft and fluctuant. Although the lesion is painless, the lesion occasionally fluctuates in size. A history of trauma was confirmed. The most likely diagnosis for this lesion is a(n):

A. fibroma
B. lymphoepithelial cyst
C. mucous retention phenomenon
D. accessory salivary gland tumor
E. bulla of pemphigoid

3. (Fig. 49-3) A 34-year-old man who is a member of the wind section of the symphony arrives at the dental clinic for evaluation of a sore lump on his palate. He states that he was unaware of the swelling until 4 days ago, when the reed of his clarinet contacted the lesion. Palpation reveals the mass to be very firm. This patient most likely has a(n):

A. periapical abscess
B. incisive canal cyst
C. necrotizing sialometaplasia
D. adenocarcinoma of the palate
E. traumatic ulcer of the palatal torus

4. (Fig. 49-4) A healthy 9-year-old male appears at the dental clinic with this soft tissue mass. It has been present for 3 weeks, but has progressively increased in size. The patient claims that moderate bleeding occurs every time he brushes, so he has avoided brushing that area for the last several days. All the adjacent teeth are asymptomatic and test vital. Periapical radiographs of the area reveal no abnormalities. This lesion shows features of malignancy.

A. true   B. false

5. (Fig. 49-4) The most likely diagnosis for the lesion described in question 4 is:

A. irritation fibroma
B. peripheral odontogenic fibroma
C. peripheral giant cell granuloma
D. peripheral fibroma with ossification
E. pyogenic granuloma

6. (Fig. 49-5) This raised soft tissue lesion is located on the patient's lower lip. In the central region of the lesion it appears translucent. Palpation reveals the lesion to be soft and fluctuant. The differential diagnosis for this lesion should include:

A. lympangioma
B. hemangioma
C. varix
D. mucocele
E. all of the above

7. (Fig. 49-5) The most likely diagnosis of this lesion is:

A. lympangioma
B. hemangioma
C. varix
D. mucocele

8. (Fig. 49-6) A 45-year-old woman appears at the dental clinic with this pink smooth-surfaced papule. It is 7mm in diameter and is firm and nonfluctant. The swelling has been present for several years and has slowly increased in size. The lesion is most likely a(n):

A. irritation fibroma
B. peripheral odontogenic fibroma
C. parulis
D. pyogenic granuloma
E. lipoma

9. (Fig. 49-7) This asymptomatic speckled red and white patch of the tongue was found in an elderly man who admitted to heavy alcohol and tobacco use. The patient was aware of the lesion's presence but was uncertain of the duration. The lesion was firm to palpation. The most likely diagnosis of this lesion is:

A. an accessory salivary gland tumor
B. traumatic erythema
C. candidiasis
D. squamous cell carcinoma
E. lichen planus

10. (Fig. 49-8) This asymptomatic lesion was discovered in a 45-year-old woman who has had several moles removed from her trunk over the last several years. The term that best describes this lesion is:

A. macule
B. papule
C. plaque
D. patch

11. (Fig. 49-8) The most likely diagnosis of this lesion is:

A. melanoplakia
B. melanotic macule
C. blue nevus
D. intramucosal nevus
E. malignant melanoma

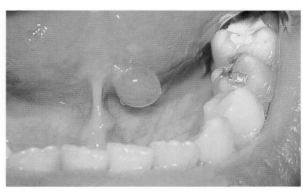

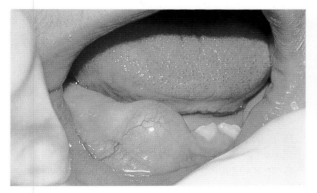

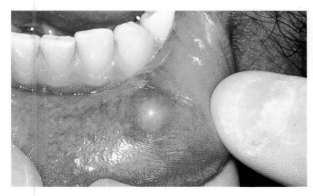

Fig. 49-1. Courtesy Dr Barney Olsen

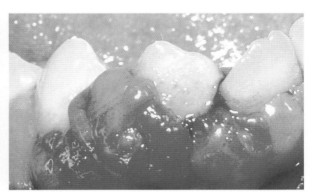

Fig. 49-2.

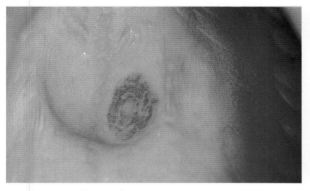

Fig. 49-3.

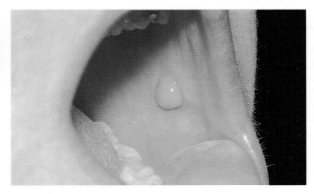

Fig. 49-4.

Fig. 49-5. Courtesy Dr Nancy Mantich

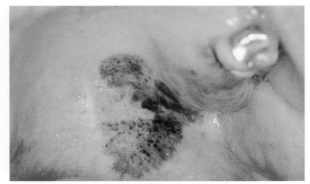

Fig. 49-6. Courtesy Dr Curt Lundeen

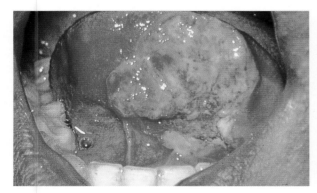

Fig. 49-7. Courtesy Dr James Cottone

Fig. 49-8. Courtesy Dr Micheal Vitt

12. (Fig. 50-1) A 66-year-old man presents to the dental clinic complaining of pain associated with these lesions on his tongue. He states that the lesions cropped up overnight and the discomfort he is experiencing is limiting his ability to swallow. Although the patient has had a history of intraoral ulcerations, he says that he has never before had one in this location. The most likely diagnosis for this condition is:

A. recurrent herpes simplex
B. aphthous stomatitis
C. traumatic ulceration
D. herpangina
E. pemphigoid

13. (Fig. 50-2) This ulcer appeared 8 days ago in a 31-year-old homosexual man following a vacation in the Carribean. He claims that the lesion began as a vesicle, but enlarged over the last several days, and is now quite painful. The regional lymph nodes on that side are tender to palpation. This lesion is most likely a:

A. traumatic ulcer
B. recurrent aphthous ulcer
C. recurrent herpetic ulcer
D. syphilitic ulcer
E. granulomatous ulcer

14. (Fig. 50-3) Two months after you treated the patient in Figure. 50-2 he returns to the dental clinic for an operative appointment. Your examination reveals scattered white plaques on the lateral border of the tongue and persistent anterior and posterior cervical lymphadenopathy. A low grade fever is also concurrent. This patient demonstrates clinical features most consistent with:

A. lichen planus
B. lupus erythematosus
C. infectious mononucleosis
D. syphilis
E. HIV infection

15. (Fig.50-3) The condition affecting this patient's tongue is most likely:

A. coated tongue
B. hairy tongue
C. hairy leukoplakia
D. leukoplakia
E. erythroleukoplakia

16. (Fig. 50-4) A 34-year-old HIV-positive man appears at the dental clinic complaining of a burning tongue. Clinical examination reveals an isolated area on the dorsal surface of the tongue that is red and denuded. Bacterial and fungal cultures are obtained. Forty-eight hours later the fun-

gal cultures are reported to be negative; the bacterial cultures are positive for gastrointestinal flora. The most likely causative organism is:

A. *Escherichia coli*
B. *Streptococcus mutans*
C. *Streptococcus viridans*
D. *Actinomyces viscosus*
E. *Treponema pallidum*

17. (Fig. 50-5) This 28-year-old woman presents to the dental clinic with the chief complaint of a "burning sensation in my mouth and throat." She has no associated complaint of dryness. Review of her medical history reveals a recent upper respiratory infection which was treated with a 14-day course of amoxicillin. Intraorally one finds multiple red patches on buccal mucosa, soft palate, and posterior pharyngeal wall that are tender to palpation. This condition is most likely:

A. lichen planus
B. pemphigoid
C. pemphigus
D. acute atrophic candidiasis
E. chronic atrophic candidiasis

18. (Fig. 50-6) These linear white plaques were discovered in a 50-year-old woman during a routine dental examination. The patient claims she has been under a lot of stress lately because of family problems. The plaques are asymptomatic and do not rub off. The most likely diagnosis is:

A. lupus erythematosus
B. lichen planus
C. candidiasis
D. frictional keratosis
E. none of the above

19. (Fig. 50-7) A 45-year-old black woman appears at the dental clinic with a swelling of the palate that has been slowly enlarging over the past several months. The lesion is painless but firm to palpation. The condition is most likely a:

A. periodontal abscess
B. palatal abscess
C. palatal torus
D. pleomorphic adenoma
E. malignant accessory salivary gland tumor

20. (Fig. 50-8) This 53-year-old woman came to the dental clinic because of burning, painful gingiva. An incisional biopsy was performed, and during the initial incision the gingiva began to slough. The biopsy report indicated that the epithelium was separating from the lamina propria below the basal cell layer. The most likely diagnosis is:

A. pemphigus
B. pemphigoid
C. lichen planus
D. lupus erythematosus
E. erythema multiforme

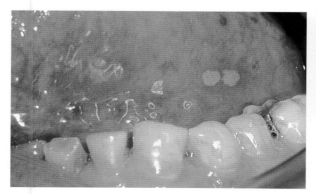

Fig. 50-1.

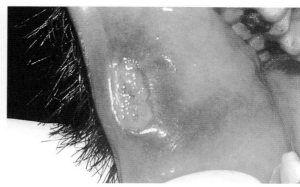

Fig. 50-2. Courtesy Dr Micheal Vitt

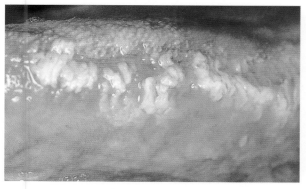

Fig. 50-3. Courtesy Dr Micheal Vitt

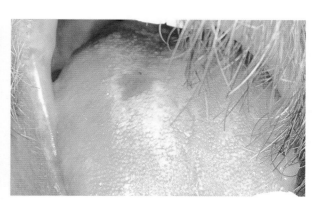

Fig. 50-4. Courtesy Dr Sol Silverman

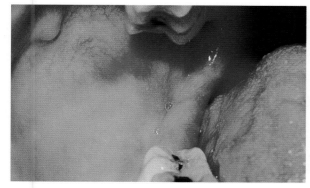

Fig. 50-5.

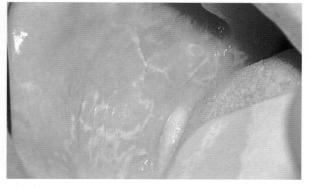

Fig. 50-6.

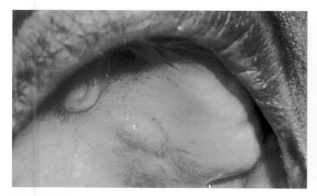

Fig. 50-7.

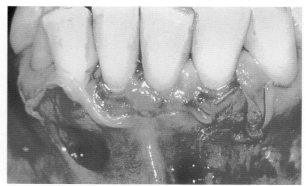

Fig. 50-8. Courtesy Dr Nancy Mantich

ANSWERS TO SELF-ASSESSMENT

1.	D	8.	A	15.	C
2.	C	9.	D	16.	A
3.	E	10.	D	17.	D
4.	B	11.	E	18.	B
5.	E	12.	B	19.	D
6.	E	13.	C	20.	B
7.	D	14.	E		

Appendix V
Glossary

Abdomen: That part of the body lying between the thorax (chest) and pelvis.

Acute: Having severe symptoms and a short course.

Adrenal gland: A small endocrine gland located near the kidney that secretes endogenous glucocorticosteroids, which control digestive metabolism; mineralocorticoids, which control sodium and potassium balance; sex hormones; and catecholamines (epinephrine and norepinephrine), which alter blood pressure and heart function.

Adrenalectomy: Surgical removal of the adrenal gland.

Afunctional: Not functioning or working.

Agenesis: Complete absence of a structure or part of a structure due to an absence of the tissue of origin in the embryo.

AIDS: Acronym for Acquired Immune Deficiency Syndrome, reserved for patients infected with HIV (Human Immunodeficiency Virus). It also refers to the terminal stage of the disease.

Allergen: A substance capable of inducing hypersensitivity or an allergic reaction.

Amalgam: An alloy used to restore teeth, composed mainly of silver and mercury.

Amelogenesis: The formation of the enamel portion of the tooth.

Amputation: Strictly, this term refers to the removal of a limb such as an arm or of an appendage such as a finger. With reference to a neuroma, however, amputation means a tumor of nerve tissue due to the severing of a nerve.

Analgesic: A drug or substance used for the relief of pain.

Analogous: Having similar properties.

Anaplastic: Pertaining to adult cells that have changed irreversibly toward more primitive cell types. Such changes are often malignant.

Anergy: A total loss of reactivity to specific antigens.

Angioma: A tumor made up of blood or lymph vessels.

Anodontia: Congenital condition in which all the teeth fail to develop.

Anomaly: Deviation from normal.

Anorexia: A lack or loss of appetite for food.

Anterior: Located toward the front (opposite of posterior).

Antibiotic: A chemical compound that inhibits the growth or replication of certain forms of life, especially pathogenic organisms such as bacteria or fungi. Antibiotics are classified as either biostatic or biocidal.

Antibiotic sensitivity: Testing a suspected organism to see if it is sensitive to destruction by one or more specific antibiotics.

Antibody: A protein produced in the body in response to stimulation by an antigen. Antibodies react specifically to antigens in an attempt to neutralize these foreign substances.

Antigen: A substance, usually a protein, that is recognized as foreign by the body's immune system and stimulates formation of a specific antibody to the antigen.

Antipyretic: A drug or substance used for the relief of fever.

Aplasia: Absence of an organ or organ part due to failure of development of the embryonic tissue of origin.

Arthralgia: Pain in one or more joints.

Aspiration: The withdrawal of fluid, usually into a syringe.

Asymptomatic: A lack of symptoms or complaints by the patient.

Atherosclerosis: A condition consisting of degeneration and hardening of the walls of arteries due to fat deposition.

Atopy: Hypersensitivity or allergy due to hereditary influences.

Atrophic: A normally developed tissue that has decreased in size.

Atypical: Pertaining to a deviation from the normal or typical state.

Autoinoculation: To inoculate with a pathogen such as a virus from one's own body. An example would be to spread herpes from your own mouth or lips to your finger.

Autosomal dominant: The appearance in offspring of one of two mutually antagonistic features in association with one of the 22 pairs of chromosomes in humans that is not concerned with sexual determination.

Bacterial plaque: A collection of bacteria, growing in a deposit of material on the surface of a tooth, that is capable of causing disease.

Bilateral: On both sides of the body.

Biopsy: Excision of living tissue for the purpose of examination by a pathologist.

Bosselated: Covered with bosses or bumps.

Bruxism: A habit related to stress or a sleep disorder, characterized by grinding one's teeth.

Bulimia: An eating disorder characterized by frequent periods of excessive food consumption followed by the purging of the ingested food by vomiting and/or the use of laxatives.

Bulla: A circumscribed, fluid-containing, elevated lesion of the skin more than 1 cm in diameter.

Carcinogen: An agent that induces cancer.

Carcinoma: A malignant growth made up of epithelial cells that are capable of infiltration and metastasis. Carcinoma is a specific form of cancer.

Cellulitis: A spreading, diffuse, edematous, and sometimes suppurative (pus-producing) inflammation in cellular tissues.

Cervical lymphadenopathy: Abnormally large lymph nodes in the neck, often caused by lymphocyte replication in response to a disease state.

Chemotaxis: Taxis or movement in response to chemical stimulation.

Chemotherapy: Treatment by chemical substances that have a specific effect on the microorganisms causing the disease. This term is usually reserved for the treatment of cancer with the use of drugs, that inhibit rapidly reproducing cells. Side effects are possible.

Chronic: Persisting over a long time; when applied to a disease, chronic means that there has been little change or extremely slow progression over a long period.

Cirrhosis: A chronic disease of the liver characterized by degenerative changes in the liver cells, the deposition of connective tissue, and other changes. The result is that the liver cells stop functioning and the flow of blood through the liver decreases. There are many causes of cirrhosis, including infection, toxic substances, and chronic alcohol abuse.

Clavicle: The collar bone, connecting the shoulder bone (scapula) to the chest bone (sternum).

Coagulation: The process of clotting, usually of blood. Clotting is the natural means by which a patient stops bleeding when a vessel has been severed.

Collagen: A protein present in the connective tissue of the body.

Coloboma: A developmental defect that may affect various parts of the eye, characterized by a missing part of the structure affected. For example, a coloboma of the lower eyelid means a missing part of the lower eyelid.

Commissure: The junction of the upper and lower lips at the corner of the mouth.

Complement: A series of enzymatic proteins in normal serum that, in the presence of a specific sensitizer, can destroy bacteria and other cells. C1 through C9 are the nine components of complement that combine with the antigen-antibody complex to produce lysis.

Concretion: A hardened mass such as calculus.

Concurrent: One or more conditions, events, or findings occurring at the same time.

Congenital: Present at, or existing from the time of birth.

Constitutional symptoms: Symptoms affecting the whole body, such as fever, malaise, anorexia, nausea, and lethargy.

Cornified: A process whereby a tissue has become horny or has thickened its outer coating.

Culture: The propagation of an organism in a medium conducive to growth.

Cyst: A pathologic epithelium-lined cavity, usually containing fluid or semisolid material.

Cytologic: Pertaining to the scientific study of cells.

Cytopathic: Pertaining to or characterized by pathologic changes in cells.

Debilitation: The process of becoming weakened.

Deciduous tooth: The primary dentition, or baby teeth. The normal number is 20.

Deglutition: The process of taking a substance through the mouth and throat into the esophagus. Deglutition is a stage of swallowing.

Dehydration: The removal of water from a substance. Prolonged fever and diarrhea cause dehydration.

Dental lamina: The embryonic tissue of origin of the teeth.

Developmental: Pertaining to growth to full size or maturity.

Diascopy: The examination of tissue under pressure through a transparent medium. For example suspected vascular lesions are examined by pressing a glass slide over an abnormality to see if the reddish tissue turns white. Since blood flows through vascular lesions, pressure causes them to turn white, thus helping to confirm the diagnosis.

Distal: Farthest from a point of reference. In dentistry, distal describes the surface farthest from the midline of the patient.

Dorsal: Directed toward or situated on the back surface (opposite of ventral).

Dysplasia: An abnormality of development characterized by the loss of normal cellular architecture.

Dysplastic: Pertaining to an abnormality of development. This term is often used to describe the appearance of abnormal, premalignant cells under the microscope. The cells begin to lose their normal maturation pattern, and have abnormally shaped, hyperchromatic nuclei.

Dyspnea: Labored or difficult breathing.

Ecchymoses: Large reddish-blue areas caused by the escape of blood into the tissues, commonly referred to as a bruise. Ecchymoses do not blanch on diascopy.

Ecosystem: The interaction of living organisms and non-living elements in a defined area.

Ectodermal: Pertaining to the outermost of the three primitive germ layers of an embryo. The middle layer is the mesoderm and the innermost layer is the endoderm. Ectodermal structures include the skin, hair, nails, oral mucous membrane, and the enamel of the teeth.

Ectopic: Located in an abnormal place. The ectopic tissue or structure may or may not be normal.

Edema: Abnormal amounts of fluid in the intercellular spaces, resulting in visible swelling.

Emanate: To give off or flow away from.

Embryonic: Pertaining to the earliest stage of development of an organism.

Encephalitis: Inflammation of the brain.

Endocrinopathy: A disease or abnormal state of an endocrine gland.

Endodermal: Pertaining to the innermost of the three primitive germ layers of an embryo. Endodermal structures include the epithelium of the pharynx, respiratory tract (except the nose), and the digestive tract.

Epistaxis: Bleeding from the nose.

Epithelium: The cellular makeup of skin and mucous membranes.

Epulis: A nodular of tumerous enlargement of the gingiva.

Erosion: The wearing away of teeth through the action of chemical substances, or a denudation of epithelium above the basal cell layer.

Eruption: An emergence from beneath a surface. For teeth, eruption means their growth into the oral cavity; it may also refer to the development of skin lesions.

Erythematous: Characterized by a redness of the tissue due to engorgement of the capillaries in the region. Erythematous lesions blanch on diascopy.

Erythroplastic: Characterized by a reddish appearance. This term implies abnormal tissue proliferation in the reddish area.

Eschar: A slough of epithelium often caused by disease, trauma, or chemical burn.

Esthetic: Pertaining to the appearance of oral or dental structures or the pleasing effect of dental restorations or procedures.

Etiology: The cause or causes of a disease, or the study thereof.

Everted: Folded or turned outward.

Exacerbation: An increase in severity.

Exanthematic: Characterized by the development of an eruption or rash.

Excisional biopsy: To completely remove a mass of tissue for the purpose of scientific analysis.

Exophytic: An outwardly growing lesion.

Extensor surface: Since the arms and legs can be extended or tensed by the appropriate extensor or tensor muscles, the anterior surface is referred to as the extensor surface and the posterior surface is referred to as the tensor surface.

Extirpate: To completely remove or eradicate.

Extremity: A limb of the body, for example an arm or leg.

Exudate: Material that has escaped from blood vessels into tissue or onto the surface of a tissue, usually because of inflammation.

Factitial: Self-induced, as in factitial injury.

Fascial plane: Spaces between adjacent bundles of fascia that cover muscles. Infection often spreads along these planes.

Fenestration: A perforation or opening in a tissue.

Fetor oris: An unpleasant or abnormal odor emanating from the oral cavity.

Field Cancerization: Malignant growths occurring in multiple sites of the oral cavity. Often the oral tissues have been exposed to a carcinogen for a long time.

Fissure: A narrow slit or cleft.

Fluctuant: Strictly, this term describes a palpated, wave-like motion that is felt in a fluid-containing lesion. In this text, the term is frequently used to describe a soft, readily yielding mass on palpation.

Fontanelle: One of several soft spots on the skull of infants and children where the bones of the skull have not yet completely united. In these areas the brain is covered only by a membrane beneath the skin.

Frenum: A fold of mucous membrane that limits the movement of an organ or organ part. For example, the lingual frenum limits tongue movement, and the labial frenuli limit lip movements.

Frontal bone: This bone forms the part of the skull consisting mainly of the forehead. The frontal bone corresponds to the front part of the skull and contains an air space called the frontal sinus.

Furcal: Pertaining to or associated with the part of a multirooted tooth where the roots join the crown.

Ganglion: A collection of cell bodies of neurons outside of the central nervous system. A ganglion is essentially a terminal through which many peripheral circuits connect with the central nervous system.

Gastroenterologist: A medical specialist whose field is disorders of the stomach and intestine.

Gastrointestinal: Pertaining to the stomach and intestine.

Genetic counselling: A form of patient counselling in which the transmission of inherited traits is discussed.

Gingivectomy: Surgical removal of gingival tissue.

Glaucoma: A disease of the eye characterized by increased intraocular pressure. This condition is often asymptomatic and, if not recognized or treated, leads to blindness.

Glossal: Pertaining to or associated with the tongue.

Glucose: A form of sugar that is the most important carbohydrate in the body's metabolism.

Glucosuria: The presence of an abnormal quantity of glucose in the urine. A sign of diabetes mellitus.

Granulomatous: Pertaining to a well-defined area that has developed as a reaction to the presence of living organisms or a foreign body. The tissue consists primarily of histiocytes.

Gravid: Pregnant.

Halitosis: An unpleasant odor of the breath or expired air.

Hamartoma: A tumor-like nodule consisting of a mixture of normal tissue usually present in an organ but existing in an unusual arrangement and/or an unusual site.

Hapten: An incomplete allergen. When combined with another substance to form a molecule, a hapten may stimulate a hypersensitivity or allergic reaction.

Hematopoietic: Pertaining to the production of blood or of its constituent elements. Hematopoiesis is the main function of the bone marrow.

Hematoma: A large ecchymosis or bruise caused by the escape of blood into the tissues. Hematomas are blue on the skin and red on the mucous membranes. As hematomas resolve they may turn brown, green, or yellow.

Hematuria: The presence of blood in the urine.

Hemihypertrophy: The presence of hypertrophy on one side only of a tissue or organ. For example, in facial hemihypertrophy one half of the face is visibly larger than the other.

Hemoglobin: The iron-containing pigment of the red blood cells. Its function is to carry oxygen to the tissues. One of the causes of anemia is a deficiency of iron, causing patients to look pale and feel tired.

Hemolysis: Generally speaking, this term refers to the disintegration of elements in the blood. A common form of hemolysis occurs during anemia and involves lysis or the dissolution of red blood cells.

Hemorrhage: Bleeding; the escape of blood from a severed blood vessel.

Hemostasis: The stoppage of blood flow. This can occur naturally by clotting or artificially by the application of pressure or the placement of sutures.

Hereditary: Transmitted or transmissible from parent to offspring; determined genetically.

Hiatal hernia: Protrusion of any structure through the hiatus of the diaphragm. Affected patients are prone to indigestion.

Histiocyte: A large phagocytic cell from the reticuloendothelial system. The reticuloendothelial system is a network made up of all of the phagocytic cells in the body, which include macrophages, Kupffer cells in the liver, and the microglia of the brain.

Histology: The microscopic study of the structure and form of the various tissues making up a living organism.

Hyperdontia: A condition or circumstance characterized by one or more extra, or supernumerary teeth.

Hyperemia: The presence of excess blood in a tissue area.

Hyperglycemia: The presence of excessive sugar or glucose in the bloodstream.

Hypermenorrhea: Excessive uterine bleeding of unusually long duration at regular intervals.

Hyperorthokeratosis: Keratin is the outermost layer of epithelium as seen under the microscope and is seen in two forms: orthokeratin and parakeratin. Orthokeratin has no visible nuclei within the outer layer, whereas in parakeratin nuclei are present. Hyperorthokeratosis is the presence of excess orthokeratin.

Hyperplasia: An increase in the size of a tissue or organ due to an increase in the *number* of constituent cells.

Hypersensitivity: Generally this term means an abnormal sensitivity to a stimulus of any kind. The term, however, is often used with specific reference to some form of allergic response.

Hypertension: High blood pressure.

Hypertrophy: An increase in the *size* of a tissue or organ due to an increase in the size of constituent cells.

Hypocalcification: Less than normal amount of calcification.

Hypodontia: The congenital absence of one or several teeth as a result of agenesis.

Hypoplasia: Incomplete development of a tissue or organ; a tissue reduced in size because of a decreased number of constituent cells.

Hypopyon: Pus in the anterior chamber of the eye.

Hypotension: Low blood pressure.

Ileum: The distal or terminal portion of the small intestine, ending at the cecum, which is a blind pouch forming the proximal or first part of the large intestine.

Ilium: The lateral or flaring part of the pelvic bone, otherwise known as the hip.

Incisional biopsy: The removal of a portion of suspected abnormal tissue for microscopic study.

Incisive papilla: A slightly elevated papule of normal tissue on the palate in the midline immediately posterior to the central incisors. Immediately beneath this structure lies the incisive canal.

Induration: Characterized by being hard; an abnormally hard portion of a tissue with respect to the surrounding similar tissue; often used to describe the feel of locally invasive malignant tissue on palpation.

Infant: A human baby from birth to two years of age.

Infarct: A localized area of ischemic necrosis resulting from a blockage of the arterial supply or the venous drainage of tissue. Ischemic necrosis is dead tissue resulting from an inadequate blood supply. An example is a heart attack, which is an infarct of heart muscle.

Insulin: A protein hormone secreted by the islands of Langerhans of the pancreas; insulin deficiency produces hyperglycemia, otherwise known as diabetes mellitus.

Invaginate: To fold and grow within, in the manner of a pouch.

Iris: The iris is the part of the eye which is blue, grey, green or brown. It is a muscular tissue and its function is to constrict and dilate the pupil. The pupil is the black portion in the middle of the iris that allows light into the eye.

Iritis: Inflammation of the iris which is often caused by viral infection or rheumatoid disease. The main symptom of iritis is photophobia (aversion to light).

Ischemia: A deficiency of blood to a body part, usually due to constriction or blockage of a blood vessel.

Kaposi's sarcoma: A malignant tumor of vascular tissue. Once rare in the Americas, it is now seen frequently in patients with AIDS. The lesions are red-purple in appearance and may be seen anywhere on the skin, especially on the face and in the oral cavity.

Keratinization: The formation of microscopic fibrils of keratin in the keratinocytes (keratin-forming cells). In the oral cavity the term is used to describe changes in the outer layer of the epithelium.

Keratotic: A condition of the skin characterized by the presence of horny growths. On the oral mucous membrane, keratotic tissue usually looks white; the term implies a thickening of the outer layer of the oral epithelium.

Lamina propria: The layer of connective tissue immediately beneath the epithelium of the oral mucosa.

Laryngeal: Pertaining to the larynx, which is a part of the airway. It is located between the pharynx at the back of the oral cavity and the trachea at the beginning of the lungs. The larynx contains the vocal cords, which make audible sounds.

Lateral: Pertaining to or situated at the side.

Leptomeninges: The two more delicate components of the meninges, the pia mater and the arachnoid.

Lesion: A site of structural or functional change in body tissues that is produced by disease or injury.

Leukoplakia: A white patch that cannot be rubbed off and that does not clinically represent any other condition.

Lipid: Fat or fatty; a naturally occurring substance made up of fatty acids.

Lobulated: Made up of lobules, which are smaller divisions of lobes. Many structures are divided into lobes and lobules, such as the brain, lung, and salivary glands. Some pathologic lesions are described as lobulated when the lesion is divided into smaller parts.

Lymphadenitis: Inflammation of lymph nodes generally resulting in enlargement and tenderness.

Lymphoblastic: Pertaining to a cell of the lymphocytic series; the term implies proliferation. Lymphoblastic is one of the forms of leukemic cancer of the white blood cells characterized by the presence of malignant lymphoblasts or immature lymphocytes.

Lymphocyte: A variety of leukocyte or white blood cell that is important to the immune reponse and that arises in the lymph nodes. Lymphocytes can be large or small, and are round, nongranular, and classified as either T- or B-lymphocytes.

Macrocheilia: Abnormally large lips.

Macrodontia: Teeth that are considerably larger than normal.

Macule: A spot or stain on the skin or mucous membrane that is neither raised nor depressed. Some examples of macules include café au lait spots, hyperemia, erythema, petechiae, ecchymoses, purpura, oral melanotic macules, and many others illustrated in this atlas.

Malaise: A constitutional symptom that describes a feeling of uneasiness, discomfort, or indisposition.

Malignant: A neoplastic growth that is not usually encapsulated, grows rapidly, and can readily metastasize.

Mastication: Chewing.

Medial: Situated toward the midline (opposite of lateral).

Melena: Darkened or black feces that are due to the presence of blood pigments; a sign of intestinal bleeding.

Meningitis: Inflammation of the meninges, which are the three membranes covering the brain and spinal cord (the dura mater, arachnoid, and pia mater). Meningitis produces both motor and mental signs such as difficulty in walking and confusion.

Mesenchymal: The meshwork of embryonic connective tissue in the mesoderm that gives rise to the connective tissue of the body, blood vessels, and lymph vessels.

Mesial: Toward the front, anterior, or midline. The mesial surface of teeth is the side of the tooth closest to the midline. The five surfaces of teeth are mesial, distal, occlusal or incisal, labial or facial, and lingual or palatal.

Metastasize: To spread or travel from one part of the body to another; a term usually reserved to describe the spread of malignant tumors.

Microdontia: Teeth that are considerably smaller than normal.

Mineralized: Characterized by the deposition of mineral, often calcium and other organic salts in a tissue. The term "calcified" is used when the mineral content is known to be calcium, whereas the term "mineralized" is more general and does not specify the exact nature of the mineral.

Monocytic leukemia: Leukemia is cancer of the white blood cells; in this instance the predominating leukocytes, or white blood cells, are monocytes.

Morphology: Descriptive of shape, form, or structure, or the science thereof.

Mucopurulent: Consisting of both mucous and pus.

Mutagenesis: The induction of genetic mutation.

Myelogenous leukemia: Leukemia is cancer of the white blood cells; in this instance the predominating leukocytes, or white blood cells, are myeloid or granular (polymorphonuclear leukocytes).

Nasopharyngitis: Inflammation of the nasopharynx which is the back of the nasal complex and upper throat. Sore throat, post-nasal drip, and fever are common signs.

Neocapillary: New growth of capillaries, which are the smallest blood vessels and connect small arterioles to small venules.

Necrosis: The death of a cell as a result of injury or disease.

Neoplasia: Characterized by the presence of new and uncontrolled cellular growth.

Neoplasm: A mass of newly formed tissue; a tumor.

Neurogenic: Originating in or from nerve tissue.

Neuropathy: Any abnormality of nerve tissue.

Neutrophil: A medium-sized white blood cell with a nucleus consisting of three to five lobes and a cytoplasm containing small granules; one of a group of white blood cells called granulocytes, the others being eosinophils and basophils. Neutrophils make up about 65% of the white blood cells in normal blood. Also known as polymorphonuclear leukocyte, PMN, or "poly."

Neutrophil chemotaxis: Taxis or movement of neutrophils in response to chemical substances or agents.

Nevus: A small tumor of the skin containing aggregations or theques of nevus cells; a mole. It may be flat or elevated, pigmented or non-pigmented, and may or may not contain hair.

Nodule: A circumscribed, usually solid lesion having the dimension of depth. Nodules are less than 1 cm in diameter.

Noncaseating: A tissue-degenerative process that forms a dry, shapeless mass resembling cheese.

Occipital bone: One of the bones that make up the skull; a thick bone at the back of the head.

Oligodontia: Presence of fewer than the normal number of teeth.

Oncogenic: Capable of causing tumor formation.

Opportunistic microorganism: Microorganisms that usually aren't pathogenic, but become so under certain circumstances, such as an environment altered by the action of antibiotics or long term steroid therapy. Opportunistic microorganisms cause opportunistic infections.

Organism: Any viable life form, such as animals, plants, and microorganisms, including bacteria, fungi, and viruses.

Otorhinolaryngologist: An ear, nose, and throat specialist.

Palliative: Treatment or the relief of symptoms, not the cause of a condition.

Pallor: Paleness of the skin or mucous membrane; an absence of a healthy color. This sign often accompanies constitutional symptoms and anemia.

Palpate: To feel with the fingers or hand.

Papule: A small mass, without the dimension of depth, that is smaller than 1 cm in diameter. When described as pedunculated, a papule is on a stalk; when described as sessile, a papule is attached at its base and does not have a stalk.

Parturition: The delivery of the fetus from the mother; to give birth.

Patch: Similar to a macule but larger; a large stain or spot, usually neither raised or depressed, which may be textured.

Patent: The condition of being open; this term is often applied to ducts, vessels, and passages to indicate that they are not blocked.

Pathognomonic: Uniquely distinctive of a specific disease or condition; usually consists of signs or findings that when present and recognized, enable the diagnosis to be made.

Pathologic: Pertaining to or caused by disease.

Pathosis: An abnormal state or condition.

Parietal bone: One of the bones that makes up the skull; there is one parietal bone on each side of the skull, forming the skull's top and upper sides.

Pedunculated: A tissue mass originating by a stalk from its base.

Periapical: Pertaining to or located at the apex (root end) of a tooth.

Perifurcal: Pertaining to or located at the furcum of a tooth; below the CEJ where the roots fuse together.

Perilabial: Pertaining to the region around or near the lips.

Perineum: The lower surface of the trunk; when a patient is lying down with legs spread apart, the perineum is the area from the base of the spine to the anal region to the genital area and, finally, to the crest of the mons pubis.

Perioral: In the proximity of or around the oral cavity.

Periorbital: In the proximity of or around the orbit, which is the bony socket of the eye.

Peripheral: Pertaining to the outer part, such as the edge or margin.

Permanent dentition: Succedaneous (adult) teeth, which follow the primary teeth. Since there are no replacements for the permanent teeth, they must last a lifetime. There are 32 permanent teeth.

Petechiae: Little red spots, ranging in size from pinpoint to several millimeters in diameter. Petechiae consist of extravasated blood.

Physiologic: Refers to normal body function (opposite of pathologic).

Pilocarpine: A drug used to stimulate salivary flow or to produce constriction of the pupil of the eye.

Plaque: An area with a flat surface and raised edges.

Platelet: One of the elements found in circulating blood. A platelet has a circular or disk-like shape and is small; hence the term platelet. Platelets aid in blood coagulation and clot retraction.

Polydipsia: Excessive thirst. A sign of disease.

Polypoid: A polyp-like protruding growth with a base that is equal in diameter to the surface of the mucosal lesion.

Polyuria: Excessive amounts of urine. A sign of disease.

Posterior: Directed toward or situated at the back (opposite of anterior).

Primary tooth: Deciduous (baby) tooth; there are 20 primary teeth.

Prognathism: A developmental deformity of the mandible that causes it to protrude abnormally.

Pruritis: Itching.

Pseudohyphae: Long, filamentous forms that can be seen under the microscope when *Candida albicans,* a fungal microorganism, assumes its pathogenic form.

Pulse: A patient's heartbeat, as felt through palpation of a blood vessel.

Punctate: Spotted; characterized by small points or punctures.

Purpuric: Pertaining to purpura, which are large bruises consisting of blood extravasated into the tissues. Bruises are bluish-purple in color.

Purulent: Containing pus.

Pustule: A well-circumscribed, pus-containing lesion, usually less than 1 cm in diameter.

Qualitative: Of or pertaining to quality; descriptive information about what something looks and feels like.

Quantitative: Of or pertaining to quantity; descriptive information about how much of something there is or how big something is.

Radiation: In dentistry, electromagnetic energy or x-rays transmitted through space. Radiation also means divergence from a common center; one of the properties of x-rays is that, like a beam of light, they diverge from their source.

Radiotherapy: Radiation therapy; the use of radiation from various sources to treat or cure malignant disorders.

Recrudescence: Recurrence of signs and symptoms of a disease after temporary abatement.

Refractory: Not readily responsive to treatment.

Remission: Improvement or abatement of the symptoms of a disease; the period during which symptoms abate.

Retinopathy: A disease or abnormality of the retina of the eye. The retina cannot be seen without special instruments, and is that part of the eye which receives and transmits visual information coming in from the pupil and lens onto the brain via the optic nerve.

Renal Failure: Inability of the kidneys to function properly. A patient whose kidneys fail completely will die without renal dialysis or a kidney transplant. One of the causes of kidney failure is prolonged hypertension (high blood pressure).

Sarcoma: A malignant growth of cells of embryonic connective tissue origin. This condition is highly capable of infiltration and metastasis.

Sarcomatous: Pertaining to sarcoma, which is a malignant tumor of mesenchymal tissue origin.

Scar: A mark or cicatrix remaining after the healing of a wound or other morbid process.

Sclera: The strong outer tunic of the eye, or whites of the eyes. When the sclera turns blue or yellow, it is a sign of systemic abnormality.

Sepsis: A morbid state resulting from the presence of pathogenic microorganisms, usually in the bloodstream.

Septicemia: The presence of pathogenic bacteria in the blood.

Sequestration: Abnormal separation of a part from the whole, such as when a piece of bone sequestrates from the mandible because of osteomyelitis; the act of isolating a patient.

Serpiginous: Characterized by a wavy or undulating margin.

Serum: The watery fluid remaining after coagulation of the blood. If clotted blood is left long enough, the clot shrinks and the fibrinogen is depleted, the remaining fluid is the serum.

Sessile: Attached to a surface on a broad base; does not have a stalk.

Sign: An objective finding or observation made by the examiner of which the patient may be unaware or does not complain.

Sinus: An airspace inside the skull, such as the maxillary sinus; an abnormal channel, fistula, or tract allowing the escape of pus.

Supernumerary: In excess of the regular number.

Splenic: Of or pertaining to the spleen, which is a structure in the upper left abdomen just behind and under the stomach. The spleen contains the largest collection of reticuloendothelial cells in the whole body; its functions include blood formation, blood storage, and blood filtration.

Spontaneous: Occurring unaided or without apparent cause; voluntary.

Superficial: Located on or near the surface.

Symptom: A manifestation of disease of which the patient is usually aware and frequently complains.

Syndrome: A combination of signs and symptoms occurring commonly enough to constitute a distinct clinical entity.

Taurodont: A malformed multirooted tooth characterized by an altered crown-to-root ratio, the crown being of normal length, the roots being abnormally short, and the pulp chamber being abnormally large.

Telangiectasia: The formation of capillaries near the surface of a tissue. Telangiectasia may be a sign of hereditary disorder, alcohol abuse, or malignancy in the region.

Template bleeding time: The amount of time necessary for bleeding to stop, following a skin incision of consistent length and depth.

Texture: Pertains to the characteristics of the surface of an area or lesion. Some descriptions of texture are as follows: smooth, rough, lumpy, and vegetative. The tiny bumps on the surface of a wart cause it to have a vegetative texture.

Therapeutic: Of or pertaining to therapy or treatment; beneficial. Therapy has as its goal the elimination or control of a disease or other abnormal state.

Thorax: That part of the body between the neck and abdomen, enclosed by the spine, ribs, and sternum. In the vernacular, the thorax is referred to as the chest. The main contents of the thorax are the heart and lungs.

Thrombophlebitis: The development of venous thrombi in the presence of inflammatory changes in the vessel wall.

Thrombosis: Formation of thrombi within the lumen of the heart or a blood vessel. A lumen is the space within a passage; a thrombus is a solid mass that can form within the heart or blood vessels from constituents in the circulating blood. Patients prone to the formation of thrombi are placed on anticoagulant therapy.

Tooth bud: The embryonic tissue of origin of the teeth; tooth buds develop from the more primitive tissue of the dental lamina.

Torus: A bony nodule on the hard palate or on the lingual aspect of the premolars.

Tourniquet test: When pressure is applied to the blood vessels of the upper arm, using a blood pressure cuff, a bleeding tendency is detected when petechiae develop in the region.

Transient: Temporary; of short duration.

Translucent: Somewhat penetrable by rays of light.

Trauma: A wound or injury; damage produced by an external force.

Trismus: Tonic contraction of the muscles of mastication; commonly referred to as lockjaw. Trismus is caused by oral infections, salivary gland infections, tetanus, trauma and encephalitis.

Trunk: The main part of the body, to which the limbs are attached. The trunk consists of the thorax and abdomen, and contains all of the internal organs. This term is also used to describe the main part of a nerve or blood vessel.

Tumor: A solid, raised mass that is larger than 1 cm in diameter and has the dimension of depth. This term also describes a mass consisting of neoplastic cells.

Ulcer: Loss of surface tissue due to a sloughing of necrotic inflammatory tissue; the defect extends into the underlying lamina propria.

Unilateral: Affecting only one side of the body.

Uremia: A toxic condition caused by the accumulation of nitrogenous substances in the blood that are normally eliminated in the urine.

Urticaria: A vascular reaction of the skin characterized by the appearance of slightly elevated patches that are either more red or paler than the surrounding skin. Urticaria is also known as hives, and may be caused by allergy, excitement, or exercise. These patches are sometimes intensely itchy.

Vasoconstriction: To diminish the diameter or caliber of a blood vessel.

Ventral: Directed toward or situated on the belly surface (opposite of dorsal).

Vermilion: That part of the lip which has a naturally pinkish red color and is exposed to the extraoral environment. The vermilion contains neither sweat glands nor accessory salivary glands.

Vermilion border: The mucocutaneous margin of the lip.

Vermilionectomy: Surgical removal of the vermilion border of the lip.

Vertigo: An unpleasant sensation characterized mainly by a feeling of dizziness or that one's surroundings are spinning or moving.

Vesicle: A well-defined lesion of the skin and mucous membranes that resembles a sac, contains fluid, and is less than 1 cm in diameter.

Visceral: Pertaining to body organs.

Viscous: Thick or sticky.

Wheal: A localized area of edema on the skin. Usually the area is raised, smooth-surfaced and is often very itchy.

Xerostomia: Dry mouth.

Index

Page numbers in italics indicate illustrations.

ectodermal, 14
epithelial, 62
in erythroplakia, 62
in leukoplakia, 62
otodental, 14

Ecchymoses, 58, *59*
Ectodermal dysplasia, 14, 46
Ectopic geographic tongue, 46
Edema, angioneurotic, 30, *31*
EES (erythromycin ethylsuccinate), 123
Elderly, actinic cheilitis in, 34
    adenoid cystic carcinoma in, 38
    angular cheilitis in, 34
    attrition in, 18
    benign lymphoid hyperplasia in, 36
    cigarette keratosis in, 56, 127
    erythema multiforme in, 90
    gingival carcinoma in, 20
    granulomatous ulcer in, 98
    herpes zoster in, 86
    lingual varicosity in, 42
    primary lymphoma of the palate in, 38
    squamous cell carcinoma in, 62
    verrucous carcinoma in, 56, 128
"Electric shock," 80
Electrogalvanic white lesion(s), 64, *65*, 130
Empirin, 115
Enamel hypoplasia, 16, *17*
Encephalitis, 84
Encephalotrigeminal angiomatosis, 60
Enisyl, 121
Enterobacter, 122
Ephelis(ides), 70, *71*, 132
Epidermal cyst(s), multiple, 14
Epidermolysis bullosa, 4
Epithelial dysplasia, 62
Epithelial inclusion cyst(s), 32
Epstein Barr virus, 44, 84, 102, 106
Epstein's pearls, 8, *9*
Epulis, congenital, 8, *9*
Epulis fissuratum, 22, *23*
Erosion, 2, *3*, 18, *19*
Erosive lichen planus, 64, *65*
Eruption cyst(s), 4
Eruption hematoma(s), 8
Erythema migrans, 46, *47*
Erythema multiforme, 90, *91*, 137
Erythematous candidiasis, 104
Erythroleukoplakia, 62, *63*, 130
Erythromycin, 123
Erythromycin ethylsuccinate, 123
Erythroplakia, 20, 62, *63*, 130
Escherichia coli, 104, 122
Exfoliative cheilitis, 2, 34, *35*
Exostosis(es), 78, *79*, 134

Fellatio syndrome, 102
Ferrous sulfate, 119
Fibroma(s), irritation, 80, *81*, 134
    occurrences of, 4, 14
    peripheral fibroma with calcification, 20, *21*
    peripheral odontogenic fibroma, 80, *81*
    traumatic, 102
Fibromatosis gingivae, hereditary, 24, *25*
Field cancerization, 62, *63*
Filiform papilla(e), 42
Fissural caries, 18
Fissure, 2, *3*
Fissured tongue, 46

Flagyl, 123
Floor of the mouth. *See* Mouth
Fluocinonide gel, 116
Fluoride therapy, 118
Fluorosis, 16
Flurazepam, 122
"Focal argyrosis," 70, *71*
Focal epithelial hyperplasia, 82, 106
"Focal gingival fibromatosis," 24
Foliate papilla(e), 42, *43*
Folic acid, 119
Follicular lymphoid hyperplasia, 36
Fordyce's granule(s), 52, *53*, 127
Freckle(s), 70, *71*, 80
Frictional keratosis, 54, *55*
Fungal infection(s), in HIV infections and
    AIDS, 104, *105*
Fungiform papilla(e), 42
Furosemide, 66
Fusion, 12, *13*
Fusobacterium, 26

Gardner's syndrome, 14, *15*, 78
"Garment trunk" nevus(i), 72
Gemination, 12, *13*
Generalized anaphylaxis, 88
Generalized fibromatosis gingivae, 24
Generalized gingival enlargement(s), drug-
        induced gingival hyperplasia, 24, *25*
    gingival edema of hypothyroidism, 24, *25*
    hereditary fibromatosis gingivae, 24, *25*
    mouthbreathing, 24, *25*
Genital herpes, 84
Genital lesion(s), 90
Genital ulcer(s), 96
Gentamycin, 124
Geographic stomatitis, 46
Geographic tongue, 46, *47*
Geotrichosis, 104
Gigantism, 12
Gingival bleeding, spontaneous, 28, *29*
Gingival carcinoma, 20, *21*
Gingival edema of hypothyroidism, 24, *25*
Gingival enlargement(s), generalized, 24, *25*
Gingival eruption cyst, 8, *9*
Gingival hyperplasia, drug-induced, 24, *25*
Gingival lesion(s), localized, 20, *21*, 22, *23*
Gingivitis, actinomycotic, 26
    acute gingivitis, 26
    acute necrotizing ulcerative gingivitis, 26, *27*,
        104
    chronic gingivitis, 26, *27*
    desquamative gingivitis, 64, 92
    diabetic gingivitis, 26, *27*
    gingivitis, 26, *27*
    HIV gingivitis, 26, 104, *105*
    hormonal gingivitis, 26, *27*
    human immunodeficiency virus (HIV)
        gingivitis, 26
    leukemic gingivitis, 26, 28, *29*
    local gingivitis, 26
    marginal gingivitis, 26, *27*
    papillary gingivitis, 26
    plasma cell gingivitis, 26, 88
    psoriasiform gingivitis, 26
    scorbutic gingivitis, 26
Gingivostomatitis, primary herpetic, 84, *85*
Glaucoma, 60
Glossitis, median rhomboid, 104, *105*
Glossodynia, 46
Glossopyrosis, 46

Gold, 66
Gonococcal pharyngitis, 102
Granular cell myoblastoma(s), 48
Granular cell tumor(s), 4, 48, *49*
Granuloma, peripheral giant cell granuloma, 20,
    21
    pyogenic granuloma, 20, *21*
Granulomatous ulcer(s), 98, *99*, 139
Graphite pencil wound(s), 70
Griseofulvin, 66
Gum boil(s), 8, 22

Hairy leukoplakia, 44, *45*, 104, 106, *107*
Hairy tongue, 44, *45*
Halcion, 122
Hand-foot-and-mouth disease, 86, *87*, 136
Heavy metal pigmentation, 74, *75*, 133
Heck's disease, 82, 106
Hemangioendothelioma, 58
Hemangioma(s), 58, *59*, 129
Hemangioma(s), macular, 60
Hematologic abnormality(ies), 66
Hematoma(s), 58, *59*
Hemihypertrophic tongue, *45*
Hemihypertrophy, 12
Hemophilus influenzae, 122
Hemostatic disorder(s), 58
Heparin, 58
Hepatomegaly, 66
"Herald spot(s)," 86
Hereditary fibromatosis gingivae, 24, *25*
Hereditary hemorrhagic telangiectasia, 60, *61*,
    129
Hereditary intestinal polyposis, 74
Herpangina, 84, *85*, 136
Herpes labialis, recurrent, 84, *85*, 106, *107*
Herpes simplex, recurrent, 84, *85*, 136
Herpes simplex virus (HSV), 2, 4, 62, 84, 90,
    98, 102, 106, *107*
Herpes virus recrudescence, 104
Herpes virus(es), 106, *107*
Herpes zoster, 4, 86, *87*, 136
Herpetic gingivostomatitis, primary, 84, *85*
Herpetic vesicle(s), 84, *85*
Herpetic whitlow, 84, *85*
Herpetiform ulceration, 94, 96, *97*, 139
Hiatal hernia, erosion due to, 18
Histoplasmosis, 98, 104, 139
HIV. *See* Human immunodeficiency virus (HIV)
HIV gingivitis, 104
HIV periodontitis, 104
"Hives," 88
Hodgkin's (disease) lymphoma, 38
Hormonal gingivitis, 26, *27*
"Hormonal tumor(s)," 20
HPV. *See* Human papilloma virus (HPV)
HSV. *See* Herpes simplex virus (HSV)
Human herpes virus VI, 84
Human immunodeficiency virus (HIV), 44, 104-
    107, *105*, *107*
Human immunodeficiency virus (HIV)
    gingivitis, 26, 104, *105*
Human immunodeficiency virus (HIV)
    periodontitis, 104, *105*
Human papilloma virus (HPV), 62, 82, 102,
    106
Hydralazine, 66
Hydrocortisone acetate ointment, 116
Hydroxyzine, 116
Hyperdontia, 14, *15*
Hyperemia, 68

Plicated tongue, 42
Plumbism, 74
Plunging ranula(e), 40
PMNR. *See* Periadenitis mucosa necrotica
    recurrens (PMNR)
PMNs. *See* Polymorphonuclear neutrophils
    (PMNs)
Polymorphonuclear neutrophils (PMNs), 28
Polyp(s), multiple intestinal polyps, 14
    pulp polyp, 18, *19*
"Port-wine stain(s)," 60
"Postherpetic neuralgia," 86
Prednisone, 117
Pregnancy, erosion due to, 18
    pyogenic granulomas during, 20
    rubella during, 14
Pregnancy gingivitis, 26, *27*
Pregnancy tumor(s), 4, 20, *21*
Primary herpetic gingivostomatitis, 84, *85*, 136
Primary lymphoma of the palate, 38, *39*
Primary syphilis, 102, *103*
Procainamide, 66
Procardia, 24
Promethazine HCl, 115
Pseudoaphtha(e), 94
Pseudoaphthous ulcer(s), 94, *95*, 138
Pseudomembranous candidiasis, 104, *105*
Psoriasiform gingivitis, 26
Pulp polyp(s), 18, *19*
Pulpitis, chronic hyperplastic, 18, 19
Purpura, 58, *59*, 129
    thrombocytopathic, 28
    thrombocytopenic, 28, *29*
Pustule(s), 4, *5*
Pyogenic granuloma, 20, *21*

Quinidine, 66
Quiz, 142-146

Radiation, 14, 18, 46
Radicular cyst(s), 4
Radicular dentin dysplasia, 16
"Rampant caries," 18
Ramsay Hunt syndrome, 86
Ranula(e), 40, *41*
RAS. *See* Recurrent aphthous stomatitis (RAS)
Recurrent aphthous stomatitis (RAS), 94, *95*,
    138
Recurrent herpes labialis, 84, *85*, 106, *107*
Recurrent herpes simplex (RHS), 84, *85*, 136
Recurrent herpetic stomatitis, 84
Recurrent scarring aphthous ulcer, 96
Red lesion(s), acute atrophic candidiasis, 68, *69*
    angular cheilitis, 68, *69*
    chronic atrophic candidiasis, 68, *69*
    chronic keratotic candidiasis, 68, *69*
    diagnosis and treatment of, 129-131
    erythroleukoplakia, 62, *63*, 130
    erythroplakia, 62, *63*, 130
    hemangioma, 58, *59*, 129
    hereditary hemorrhagic telangiectasia, 60, *61*,
        129
    lichen planus, 64, *65*, 130
    lichenoid drug eruption, 66, *67*
    lupus erythematosus, 66, *67*, 130
    lupus-like drug eruption, 66, *67*
    purpura, 58, *59*, 129
    squamous cell carcinoma, 62, *63*, 130, 139
    Sturge-Weber syndrome, 60, *61*, 129
    thrombus, 58, *59*, 129

varicosity, 58, *59*, 129
Red/white lesion(s), acute atrophic candidiasis,
    68, *69*
    acute pseudomembranous candidiasis, 68, *69*
    angular cheilitis, 68, *69*
    chronic atrophic candidiasis, 68, *69*
    chronic keratotic candidiasis, 68, *69*
    diagnosis and treatment of, 130-131
    electrogalvanic white lesion, 64, *65*, 130
    erythroleukoplakia, 62, *63*, 130
    erythroplakia, 62, *63*, 130
    lichen planus, 64, *65*, 130
    lichenoid drug eruption, 66, *67*, 131
    lupus erythematosus, 66, *67*, 130
    lupus-like drug eruption, 66, *67*, 131
Restoril, 122
Reticular lichen planus, 64, *65*
Retrocuspid papilla, 78, *79*, 134
Reye's syndrome, 86
Rheumatoid arthritis, 66
RHS. *See* Recurrent herpes simplex (RHS)
Rieger's syndrome, hypodontia in, 14
"Root caries," 18
"Rootless teeth," 16
Rubella during pregnancy, 14
Rx abbreviation(s), 111

Saliva substitute, 120
Salivart, 120
Salivary calculi, 40, *41*
Salivary gland neoplasia, 32
    benign, 38, *39*
        monomorphic adenoma, 38, 39
        pleomorphic adenoma, 38, 39
    malignant, 38, *39*
        adenoid cystic carcinoma, 38, 39
        mucoepidermoid carcinoma, 38, 39
Salivary gland tumor(s), accessory, 32, *33*
Scalloped tongue, 44, *45*
Scar, 2, *3*, 54, *55*
Scarifying stomatitis, 96
Scorbutic gingivitis, 26
Scrotal tongue, 42
Secondary syphilis, 102, *103*
Sedative/hypnotics, 122
Seldane, 120
Self-assessment quiz, 142-146
Sexually related and infectious condition(s),
        acquired immune deficiency syndrome
        (AIDS), 104-107, *105t*, *107*
    HIV infection, 104-107, *105*, *107*
    infectious mononucleosis, 102, *103*
    sexually transmitted pharyngitis, 102, *103*
    syphilis, 102, *103*
    traumatic conditions, 102, *103*
Sexually transmitted pharyngitis, 102, *103*
Shingles, 2, 86
Sialolith(s), 40, *41*
Sialometaplasia, necrotizing, 38, *39*
Silver pigmentation, 74
Sinus, 2, *3*
Sjögren's syndrome, 36, 46, 66
SLE. *See* Systemic lupus erythematosus (SLE)
Smallpox, 2, 4
Smoker's melanosis, 70, *71*, 132
Smooth surface caries, 18
Snuff dipper's patch, 2, 56, *57*, 128
Snuff keratosis, 56
Speckled erythroplakia, 62, *63*, 130
Speckled leukoplakia, 62, 63
Splenomegaly, 66

Spontaneous gingival bleeding, agranulocytosis,
    28, *29*
    with cirrhosis, *29*
    with clotting-factor deficiency, *29*
    cyclic neutropenia, 28, *29*
    leukemic gingivitis, 28, *29*
    thrombocytopathic purpura, 28
    thrombocytopenic purpura, 28, *29*
Squamous cell carcinoma(s), *21*, 62, *63*, 98, *99*,
    106, 130, 139
Squamous papilloma, 4, 82, 106
Stannous fluoride, 118
Staphylococcus aureus, 34
Steroid(s), 68
Stevens-Johnson syndrome, 90, *91*, 137
Stomatitis, 90
    allergic, 88, 89
    contact, 88, 89
    denture, 68, *69*
    nicotine, 56, *57*
    scarifying stomatitis, 96
Stomatitis venenata, 88
Streptococcus, 94
Streptococcus mutans, 18
Streptococcus sanguis, 18
Streptomycin, 66, 98
Striated lichen planus, 64
Sturge-Weber syndrome, 60, *61*, 129
Subacute cutaneous lupus erythematosus, 66
Sublingual gland, mucocele of, 40
Submandibular gland, 40
Sulfa-containing drug(s), 90
Sulfamethoxazole, 122
Superficial ranula(e), 40
Supernumerary teeth, 12, 14
Sutton's disease, 96
Swelling(s) of the floor of the mouth, dermoid
        cyst, 40, *41*
    mucous retention phenomenon, 40, *41*
    ranula, 40, *41*
    salivary calculi, 40, *41*
Swelling(s) of the lip, angioedema, 30, *31*
    cellulitis, 30, *31*
    cheilitis glandularis, 30, *31*
    cheilitis granulomatosa, 30, *31*
    trauma, 30, *31*
Swelling(s) of the palate, 36, *37*, 38, *39*
Syphilis, 2, 102, *103*
Systemic lupus erythematosus (SLE), 66

"Target" lesion(s), 90
Tattoo(s), 70, *71*, 132
    amalgam, 70
Taurodontism, 16
TB. *See* Tuberculosis (TB)
Teenager(s). *See* Young adult(s)
Teeth, numbers of, 14, *15*
Teeth defect(s), acquired, 18, *19*
Teeth morphology, alterations in, 12, *13*
Teeth structure, alterations in, 16, *17*
Telangiectasia(s), 66
Telangiectasia(s), hereditary hemorrhagic, 60,
    61, 129
Temazepam, 122
Temporomandibular joint disorder(s), 44
Terephthalate, 115
Terfenadine, 120
Tertiary syphilis, *103*
Tetracycline HCl, 117
Tetracycline HCl, 123
Tetracycline(s), 68, 102

Tetracyn, 117
Thalidomide, 96
"Theque(s)," 72
Therapeutic protocol(s), analgesics, 115
  antianxiety agents, 119
  antibiotic therapy, 122-124
  anti-fungal therapy, 121
  antihistamines, 116, 120
  anti-viral therapy, 121
  fluoride therapy, 118
  immunosuppressive agents, 117
  nutrient deficiency therapy, 119
  oral antimicrobial rinses, 117
  saliva substitute, 120
  sedative/hypnotics, 122
  topical corticosteroids, 116
  topical oral anesthetics, 118
Thiazide(s), 66
Thombocytopenia, 28, 29
Thrombocytopathia, 28
Thrombocytopathic purpura, 28
Thrombocytopenic purpura, 28, 29, 58
Thrombus, 58, 59, 129
Thrush, 8, 9, 68, 69
Thyroid, lingual, 48, 49
Tobacco-associated pigmentation, 70
Tobacco-associated white lesion(s), 56, 57
Tobacco chewer's lesion(s), 56
Tongue, anemia, 46, 47
  ankyloglossia, 42, 43
  cyst of Blandin-Nuhn, 48, 49
  fissured tongue, 42, 43, 46
  geographic tongue, 46, 47
  hairy tongue, 44, 45
  hemihypertrophic tongue, 45
  lingual thyroid, 48, 49
  macroglossia, 44
  median rhomboid glossitis, 48, 49
  normal tongue anatomy, 42, 43
  scalloped tongue, 44, 45
  xerostomia, 46, 47
"Tongue-tie," 42
Tonsil, lingual, 42, 43
Tooth. See headings beginning with Teeth
"Toothbrush abrasion," 18, 19
Topical corticosteroid(s), 116
Topical oral anesthetics, 118
Torus palatinus, 36, 37
Torus(i), 78, 79, 134
"Tram-line(s)," 60
Tetracycline HCl, 123
Traumatic fibroma(s), 102
Traumatic neuroma(s), 80, 81, 135
Traumatic swelling, of lips, 30, 31
Traumatic ulcer(s), 94, 95, 102, 103, 138
Traumatic white lesion(s), 54, 55, 127
Treatment of common oral lesions, 127-139
"Trench mouth," 26
Treponema, 26
Treponema pallidum, 62, 102
Tri-Statin, 121
Triamcinolone acetonide ointment, 116
Triazolam, 122
Trimethadione, 66
Trimethoprim, 122
Trophic ulcer(s), 94
Tubercle, Leong's tubercle, 12

Tuberculosis (TB), 98, 139
Tuberous sclerosis, 80
Tumor(s), 4, 5
  accessory salivary gland tumor, 32, 33
  desmoid tumor, 14
  granular cell tumor, 48, 49
  melanotic neuroectodermal tumor of infancy,
    8, 9
  mesenchymal tumor, 32, 33
  multiple dermoid tumors, 14
Turner's teeth, 16, 17
Tylenol, 115

Ulcer(s), 2, 3
Ulcerative lesion(s), Behçet's syndrome, 96, 97,
    139
  chemotherapeutic ulcer, 98, 99, 139
  diagnosis and treatment of, 138-139
  granulomatous ulcer, 98, 99, 139
  herpetiform ulceration, 96, 97, 139
  ischemic, 94
  major aphthous stomatitis, 96, 97, 138
  pseudoaphthous ulcer, 94, 95, 138
  recurrent aphthous stomatitis, 94, 95, 138
  squamous cell carcinoma, 98, 99, 139
  traumatic ulcer, 94, 95, 138
  trophic ulcer, 94
Uremia, 28
Urticaria, 88

Valisone, 116
Valium, 119
Vancocin, 124
Vancomycin, 124
Varicella, 86, 87, 136
Varicella zoster virus (VZV), 2, 84, 106, 107
Varicosity(ies), 58, 59, 129
Varicosity(ies), lingual, 42, 43
Variola, 2
Varix(ices), 58, 59
Vascular disease, 46
Vascular hyperplasia, 60
Veillonella, 26
Venereal disease, 102
Venereal wart(s), 82
Venous dilation(s), 42
Verruca vulgaris, 106, 135
Verruca(e) vulgaris, 82, 83
Verrucous carcinoma (of Ackerman), 56, 57,
    128
Vesicle(s), 4, 5
Vesicle(s), herpetic, 84, 85
Vesiculobullous lesion(s), allergic reactions, 88,
    89, 136, 137
  benign mucous membrane pemphigoid, 92,
    93, 137
  diagnosis and treatment of, 136-137
  erythema multiforme, 90, 91, 137
  hand-foot-and-mouth disease, 86, 87, 136
  herpangina, 84, 85, 136
  herpes zoster, 86, 87, 136
  pemphigus vulgaris, 92, 93, 137
  primary herpetic gingivostomatitis, 84, 85,
    136
  recurrent herpes simplex, 84, 85, 136

Stevens-Johnson syndrome, 90, 91, 137
  varicella, 86, 87, 136
Vincent's infection, 26
Viral infection(s), in HIV infection and AIDS,
    106, 107
  ulcers and, 2
  vesicles and, 4
Von Recklinghausen's disease, 32, 80
Vulgaris, 92, 93
Vulvovaginitis, 90
VZV. See Varicella zoster virus (VZV)

Wandering rash, 46
Warfarin, 58
Wart, common. See Verruca vulgaris
  venereal. See Condyloma accuminatum
"Weeping" bulla(e), 92
"Weeping" vesiculobullous lesion(s), 90
Wharton's duct, 40
Wheal(s), 2, 3, 88
White coated tongue, 44
White lesion(s), cigarette keratosis, 56, 57, 127
  diagnosis and treatment of, 127-128
  electrogalvanic white lesion, 64, 65
  Fordyce's granules, 52, 53, 127
  frictional keratosis, 54, 55
  leukoedema, 52, 53, 127
  leukoplakia, 54, 55, 127
  linea alba buccalis, 52, 53, 127
  morsicatio buccarum, 52, 53, 127
  nicotine stomatitis, 56, 57, 128
  scar, 54, 55
  snuff dipper's patch, 56, 57, 128
  tobacco-associated white lesions, 56, 57
  traumatic white lesion, 54, 55, 127
  verrucous carcinoma (of Ackerman), 56, 57,
    128
  white sponge nevus, 54, 55, 127
White sponge nevus(i), 54, 55, 127
Whitlow, herpetic, 84, 85
Wickham's stria(e), 64

Xanax, 119
Xerolube, 120
Xerostomia, 18, 46, 47
Xylocaine, 118

Yellow hairy tongue, 44
Young adult(s), aphthae in, 94, 138
  dermoid cyst in, 40
  erythema multiforme in, 90, 137
  exfoliative cheilitis in, 34
  hand-foot-and-mouth disease in, 86, 136
  herpangina in, 84, 136
  herpes zoster in, 86
  herpetic gingivostomatitis in, 84
  infectious mononucleosis in, 102
  iron deficiency anemia in, 46
  lymphoepithelial cyst in, 78, 134
  major aphthous in, 96
  mucous retention phenomenon in, 32, 40
  Stevens-Johnson syndrome in, 90, 137
  syphilis in, 102

Zovirax, 121